CONTENTS

INTRODUCTION

What is Breville?

Breville is an Australian manufacturer of little home appliances (based in Sydney), including premium countertop ovens, non-premium ovens (like a regular toaster oven), blenders, microwaves, and also makes Nespresso coffee machines. The society was founded in 1932 and the brand name Breville was taken from the two founders' last names: Bill O'Brien and Harry Norville.

In 2002, the Breville brand was introduced to the United States, and in recent years, has introduced juicers, pressure cookers, food processors, and blenders. By 2011, sales for its juicers doubled by the U.S. following a Breville juicer featured in the Netflix series 'Fat, Sick and Nearly Dead".

The Breville Smart Oven Air

The Breville Smart Oven Air has many features similar to those of Breville's other ovens, or even a toaster oven. Breville countertops are renowned for having many features and functions. The Breville smart stainless-steel oven has features that you would expect as a slow bake and baking feature plus a couple more, including Air Fry and Dehydrate. Air frying is a healthier way to crunch your food than conventional frying oil. Air frying uses Super Convection's intelligent machine to help move air inside the oven for the best crisp. Super Convection runs the built-in convection ventilator speeds much higher than regular Convection baking. The two-speed convection fan is one of the little appliance market's only two-speed fans.

For every baking function, the Element IQ device works to optimize the heating elements, convection fan, and time to achieve each task's best results. For each mode, you can use the Element IQ program, or just manually use your oven.

The lowest-priced countertops in Breville are without convection fans. These are not convection ovens while the Breville Smart Oven Pro (the variant in price just below the Smart Air) has a convection fan but not a two-speed fan.

What are the Smart Oven Air functions?

The Smart Air has 13 pre-set features, that's quite a lot. The following functions are: bake, roast, broil, warm, pizza, proof, air fry, toast, bagel, reheat, slow bake, cookies, and dehydrating.

These pre-set functions work with the company's Element IQ System and each of the six oven heating elements to bake automatically for optimal performance. These heating elements are put on the top and bottom of the oven, and each element is turned on or off by the Element IQ System at higher or lower power, depending on the feature you select.

Learning the controls

The great thing about the Breville Smart Air Fryer Oven is that all the controls are labeled for easy use, so you don't have to bother with confusing dials.

Function knob:

This knob allows you to select which baking program you would like.

LCD Display:

Displays the number of pieces of bread, darkness setting, current time, baking temperature, and amount of time left to bake.

TEMP/DARKNESS button:

Select the TEMPERATURE or DARKNESS setting for the TOAST.

UP and DOWN selection buttons:

Use to adjust time, temperature, and amount of darkness.

TIME/SLICES button:

Use to adjust the baking time and number of slices of bread.

A BIT MORE:

This function adds a little amount of baking time. The amount of time varies depending on which baking program you have chosen.

START/CANCEL button:

It starts and stops the baking process

F/C button:

Choose Fahrenheit or Celsius.

FROZEN FOODS button:

Adds extra time to the baking process to defrost frozen foods.

How to arrange the Smart Oven before first use

It's necessary to run the smart oven empty for about 20 minutes before first taking off any protective substance stick on the elements. Before conducting the test, put the oven into the well-ventilated area and follow the instructions given below.

1.   First, take off the promotional stickers, poly covers on any packaging materials from the oven.

2.   Take off the roasting pan, crumb tray, dehydrate or air fry basket, roasting pan, pizza pan, wire rack, broiling rack, from poly packaging and wash them into warm water or soapy water using a soft cloth.

3.   Take a soft sponge to wipe the interior of the oven and dry it.

4.   Put the oven into a well-ventilated area. Make sure a minimum 4 to 6 inches of distance space on both sides of the oven.

5.   Include the crumb tray in the oven and plug the power cord into a power outlet.

6.   The oven screen will illuminate with a warning sound, and the functions menu will be displayed and the default indicator is on TOAST menu setting.

7.   Now rotate the SELECT-CONFIRM dial till the pointer is on PIZZA settings.

8.   Press the START-STOP button. Then, the button backlight will light up red and the oven digital display screen will light up orange with a "beep".

9.   Then the display indicating PRE-HEATING by blinking. After completion of pre-heating the oven sound alerts and the timers automatically begin countdowns.

10.   After finishing the baking cycle, the oven alarm sounds, then the START-STOP backlight off and the oven LCD turns on in color. This will denote that the oven is ready for first use.

How do I use my Breville Air Fryer?

As described above, the Element IQ System uses the oven's heating elements at higher or lower temperatures and turns some on or off to bake the best way you choose. Here you can know what sorts of stuff your Breville air fryer can bake with.

1.   **Roast**

Roast mode is intended for the baking of thick meat or poultry cuts. Ideally, roasting adds a crisp exterior to what you bake while leaving moist and tender inside. Note that when using Roast, use rack position 6 in the oven (the rack's location is indicated at the window of the oven to let you know where position 6 is located).

2.   **Bake**

Bake mode is designed to use heat for baking cookies, muffins, and similar food evenly in the top and bottom of your oven. Baking also works well in your included baking pan or on the wire rack with dense savory frozen dishes such as lasagna or pot-pies. Using oven rack position 6 when using Bake mode, as in Roast mode, and use the rack position indicator on the oven window to show where position 6 is located.

3.   **Broil**

Broiling is about searing the top side of your food at high temperatures. Broil mode uses the heating elements at the top of the oven to crisp open-faced sandwiches, thinly sliced beef, seafood, sausages, and vegetables at their maximum power.

4.   **Toast**

Toast is what you might anticipate, essentially baking the bread's top layer while keeping the inside soft and moist. Toast mode can also be used to heat and crisp English muffins and frozen waffles. Use oven position 4 in Toast mode. The oven suits up to 9 slices of conventionally sliced bread. Using the "Time" dial in the oven's control panel to pick the number of slices you are toasting with.

5.   **Bagel**

The Bagel mode is designed to bake the inside of a thick bagel, crumpet, or speciality bread and only toast the outside lightly. For Bagel mode, using rack position 4 (see the positions indicated on the window). The oven is designed to accommodate up to 10 slices of bagel.

6.   **Warm**

This function helps to prevent bacterial growth. It maintains your oven temperature at about 160°F.

7.   **Pizza**

This feature melts the cheese toppings and browns it even from above during crispy pizza cuts.

Proof

Utilizing this function, you can make the ideal environment for proofing doughs, rolls, pizza and bread.

8.   **Airfry**

You can prepare crispy and brown food. This feature is ideal for doing French fries.

9.   **Reheat**

This is ideal for reheat your frozen food or leftover foods without browning or drying the food.

10.   **Cookies**

This function is used for baking your favourite cookies and other baked treats.

11.   **Slow bake**

This is utilized for baking food for a long time at low temperature.

12.   **Dehydrate**

This function is used to dry out food without heating or baking them. It's ideal for dehydrating your favourite fruit slices.

What does it not do?

The Breville Smart Air Fryer Oven is a marvel of functionality. From convection baking to perfect defrosting, it does so many things. But there are also a few things it can't do.

The Breville Smart Oven will not take the put of your microwave because it will not head food as quickly. It does, however, heat up much faster than a conventional oven. You are also somewhat limited by the size of the Smart Oven.

While it does feature a big baking compartment, you will not be able to bake a twenty-pound turkey in it. Other than these few limitations, it can handle most of your baking needs.

Who is not good for?

While the Breville Smart Air Fryer Oven is perfect for nearly any situation, if you have limited space in your kitchen and do not need another baking appliance, this oven may not be for you. Also, if your family prefers only to make big meals, the Smart Oven's little size may not be big enough to meet your needs.

Benefits of Breville Smart Air Fryer Oven

Here are some benefits:

• Every heating system automatically adjusts to match your preferred setting;

• Super convection setting reduces baking time by 30% while providing perfect crispness – ensuring quick and even roasting, frying and dehydration of the air;

• The 13 pre-programmed settings include: toast, bagel, broil, bake, roast, hot, pizza, proof, air-frying, reheating, cookies, slow baking and dehydration;

• Six independent quartz heating elements transfer the power where food is most needed – above and below – resulting in an effective baking process;

• Air-frying function combines high heat and super-convection to maximize airflow, resulting in deliciously crispy food;

• PID regulation eliminates over-shooting for accurate and stable temperatures;

• A big-capacity countertop oven lets you roast a 14-lb. Turkey, toast nine slices of bread, bake a 12-cup muffin tray…

Care and cleaning

Before starting, the cleaning process makes sure that the power cord has been taken off from the power outlet. Allow the oven and accessories to cool to room temperature before starting the cleaning process.

Clean the oven body with a soft, damp sponge and use a detergent on a sponge during the cleaning process. When cleaning the glass door, you can use a glass cleaner and a plastic cleaning sponge. Do not use metal scouring pads as they could scratch the surface of the oven.

The internal body of the oven consists of a non-stick coating. Utilize a soft, damp sponge to clean the inside of the oven. Utilize the cleaner to the sponge, do not apply it directly to the oven body before cleaning the elements, make sure the oven has cooled down to room temperature, then wipe it gently with a soft damp cloth or sponge.

Clean the crumb tray with the help of a soft, damp sponge. You can use a non-abrasive liquid cleaner. Apply the cleaner to a sponge and wipe the tray.

To clean a pan, dip it in hot soapy water and wash it with a plastic sponge or soft sponge.

Always remember to dry all accessories well before placing them in the oven. Insert the crumb tray into its position before plugging the oven into its socket. The oven is ready for the next use.

APPETIZERS AND SIDE DISHES

1. Roasted Beets With Grapefruit Glaze

Servings: 5
Cooking Time: 10 Minutes
Ingredients:

- 3 pounds beets
- 1 cup fresh-squeezed grapefruit juice (approximately 2 medium grapefruits)
- 1 tablespoon rice vinegar
- 3 scant tablespoons pure maple syrup
- 1 tablespoon corn starch

Directions:

1. Start by preheating toaster oven to 450°F. Place beets in a roasting pan and sprinkle with water.
2. Roast beets until soft enough to be pierced with a fork, at least 40 minutes.
3. Remove beets and allow to cool until you can handle them.
4. Peel skin off beets and thinly slice.
5. Mix together grapefruit juice, syrup, and vinegar in a small bowl.
6. Pour corn starch into a medium sauce pan and slowly add grapefruit mixture. Stir together until there are no clumps.
7. Heat sauce to a light boil then reduce heat and simmer for 5 minutes, stirring often.
8. Drizzle glaze over beets and serve.
- **Nutrition Info:** Calories: 175, Sodium: 211 mg, Dietary Fiber: 6.0 g, Total Fat: 0.6 g, Total Carbs: 40.7 g, Protein: 4.9 g.

2. Jalapeños Peppers With Chicken & Bacon

Servings:4
Cooking Time: 40 Minutes
Ingredients:

- 8 jalapeño peppers, halved lengthwise
- 4 chicken breasts, butterflied and halved
- 6 oz cream cheese
- 6 oz Cheddar cheese
- 16 slices bacon
- 1 cup breadcrumbs
- Salt and black pepper to taste
- 2 eggs

Directions:

1. Season the chicken with salt and pepper. In a bowl, add cream cheese and cheddar cheese and mix well. Take each jalapeño and spoon in the cheese mixture to the brim. On a working board, flatten each piece of chicken and lay 2 bacon slices each on them. Place a stuffed jalapeno on each laid out chicken and bacon set, and wrap the jalapeños in them.
2. Preheat Breville on AirFry function to 350 F. Add the eggs to a bowl and pour the breadcrumbs in another bowl. Also, set a flat plate aside. Take each wrapped jalapeño and dip it into the eggs and then in the breadcrumbs. Place them on the flat plate. Lightly grease the fryer basket with cooking spray. Arrange 4-5 breaded jalapeños on the basket and press Start.
3. AirFry for 7 minutes, turn the jalapeños and cook for 4 minutes. Once ready, remove them onto a paper towel-lined plate. Serve with a sweet dip for an enhanced taste.

3. Blistered Shishito Peppers With Lime Juice

Servings:3
Cooking Time: 9 Minutes
Ingredients:

- ½ pound (227 g) shishito peppers, rinsed
- Cooking spray
- Sauce:
- 1 tablespoon tamari or shoyu
- 2 teaspoons fresh lime juice
- 2 large garlic cloves, minced

Directions:

1. Spritz the air fryer basket with cooking spray.
2. Place the shishito peppers in the basket and spritz them with cooking spray.
3. Put the air fryer basket on the baking pan and slide into Rack Position 2, select Roast, set temperature to 392ºF (200ºC), and set time to 9 minutes.
4. Meanwhile, whisk together all the ingredients for the sauce in a large bowl. Set aside.

5. After 3 minutes, remove from the oven. Flip the peppers and spritz them with cooking spray. Return to the oven and continue cooking.
6. After another 3 minutes, remove from the oven. Flip the peppers and spray with cooking spray. Return to the oven and continue roasting for 3 minutes more, or until the peppers are blistered and nicely browned.
7. When cooking is complete, remove the peppers from the oven to the bowl of sauce. Toss to coat well and serve immediately.

4. Sausage Mushroom Caps(2)

Servings: 2
Cooking Time: 20 Minutes
Ingredients:
- ½ lb. Italian sausage
- 6 large Portobello mushroom caps
- ¼ cup grated Parmesan cheese.
- ¼ cup chopped onion
- 2 tbsp. blanched finely ground almond flour
- 1 tsp. minced fresh garlic

Directions:
1. Use a spoon to hollow out each mushroom cap, reserving scrapings.
2. In a medium skillet over medium heat, brown the sausage about 10 minutes or until fully cooked and no pink remains. Drain and then add reserved mushroom scrapings, onion, almond flour, Parmesan and garlic.
3. Gently fold ingredients together and continue cooking an additional minute, then remove from heat
4. Evenly spoon the mixture into mushroom caps and place the caps into a 6-inch round pan. Place pan into the air fryer basket
5. Adjust the temperature to 375 Degrees F and set the timer for 8 minutes. When finished cooking, the tops will be browned and bubbling. Serve warm.
- **Nutrition Info:** Calories: 404; Protein: 24.3g; Fiber: 4.5g; Fat: 25.8g; Carbs: 18.2g

5. Cilantro Roasted Cauliflower(1)

Servings: 4

Cooking Time: 20 Minutes
Ingredients:
- 2 cups chopped cauliflower florets
- 1 medium lime
- 2 tbsp. chopped cilantro
- 2 tbsp. coconut oil; melted
- ½ tsp. garlic powder.
- 2 tsp. chili powder

Directions:
1. Take a large bowl, toss cauliflower with coconut oil. Sprinkle with chili powder and garlic powder. Place seasoned cauliflower into the air fryer basket
2. Adjust the temperature to 350 Degrees F and set the timer for 7 minutes
3. Cauliflower will be tender and begin to turn golden at the edges. Place into serving bowl. Cut the lime into quarters and squeeze juice over cauliflower. Garnish with cilantro.
- **Nutrition Info:** Calories: 73; Protein: 1g; Fiber: 1g; Fat: 5g; Carbs: 3g

6. Turmeric Mushroom(1)

Servings: 4
Cooking Time: 20 Minutes
Ingredients:
- 1 lb. brown mushrooms
- 4 garlic cloves; minced
- ¼ tsp. cinnamon powder
- 1 tsp. olive oil
- ½ tsp. turmeric powder
- Salt and black pepper to taste.

Directions:
1. In a bowl, combine all the ingredients and toss.
2. Put the mushrooms in your air fryer's basket and cook at 370°F for 15 minutes
3. Divide the mix between plates and serve as a side dish.
- **Nutrition Info:** Calories: 208; Fat: 7g; Fiber: 3g; Carbs: 5g; Protein: 7g

7. Jicama Fries(3)

Servings: 4
Cooking Time: 20 Minutes
Ingredients:
- 1 small jicama; peeled.
- ¼ tsp. onion powder.

- ¾ tsp. chili powder
- ¼ tsp. ground black pepper
- ¼ tsp. garlic powder.

Directions:
1. Cut jicama into matchstick-sized pieces.
2. Place pieces into a small bowl and sprinkle with remaining ingredients. Place the fries into the air fryer basket
3. Adjust the temperature to 350 Degrees F and set the timer for 20 minutes. Toss the basket two or three times during cooking. Serve warm.
- **Nutrition Info:** Calories: 37; Protein: 8g; Fiber: 7g; Fat: 1g; Carbs: 7g

8. Grilled Sandwich With Ham & Cheese

Servings: 2
Cooking Time: 15 Minutes
Ingredients:
- 4 bread slices
- ¼ cup butter
- 2 ham slices
- 2 mozzarella cheese slices

Directions:
1. Preheat Breville on AirFry function to 360 degrees F. Place 2 bread slices on a flat surface. Spread butter on the exposed surfaces. Lay cheese and ham on two of the slices.
2. Cover with the other 2 slices to form sandwiches. Place the sandwiches in the frying basket. Select Bake function, adjust the temperature to 380 F, and press Start. Cook for 5 minutes.

9. Beef Enchilada Dip

Servings: 8
Cooking Time: 10 Minutes
Ingredients:
- 2 lbs. ground beef
- ½ onion, chopped fine
- 2 cloves garlic, chopped fine
- 2 cups enchilada sauce
- 2 cups Monterrey Jack cheese, grated
- 2 tbsp. sour cream

Directions:
1. Place rack in position

2. Heat a large skillet over med-high heat. Add beef and cook until it starts to brown. Drain off fat.
3. Stir in onion and garlic and cook until tender, about 3 minutes. Stir in enchilada sauce and transfer mixture to a small casserole dish and top with cheese.
4. Set oven to convection bake on 325°F for 10 minutes. After 5 minutes, add casserole to the oven and bake 3-5 minutes until cheese is melted and mixture is heated through.
5. Serve warm topped with sour cream.
- **Nutrition Info:** Calories 414, Total Fat 22g, Saturated Fat 10g, Total Carbs 15g, Net Carbs 11g, Protein 39g, Sugar 8g, Fiber 4g, Sodium 1155mg, Potassium 635mg, Phosphorus 385mg

10. Green Beans

Servings: 4
Cooking Time: 20 Minutes
Ingredients:
- 6 cups green beans; trimmed
- 1 tbsp. hot paprika
- 2 tbsp. olive oil
- A pinch of salt and black pepper

Directions:
1. Take a bowl and mix the green beans with the other ingredients, toss, put them in the air fryer's basket and cook at 370°F for 20 minutes
2. Divide between plates and serve as a side dish.
- **Nutrition Info:** Calories: 120; Fat: 5g; Fiber: 1g; Carbs: 4g; Protein: 2g

11. Mixed Veggie Bites

Servings: 5
Cooking Time: 10 Minutes
Ingredients:
- ¾ lb. fresh spinach, blanched, drained and chopped
- ¼ of onion, chopped
- ½ of carrot, peeled and chopped
- 1 garlic clove, minced
- 1 American cheese slice, cut into tiny pieces
- 1 bread slice, toasted and processed into breadcrumbs

- ½ tablespoon corn flour
- ½ teaspoon red chili flakes
- Salt, as required

Directions:
1. In a bowl, add all the ingredients except breadcrumbs and mix until well combined.
2. Add the breadcrumbs and gently stir to combine.
3. Make 10 equal-sized balls from the mixture.
4. Press "Power Button" of Air Fry Oven and turn the dial to select the "Air Fry" mode.
5. Press the Time button and again turn the dial to set the cooking time to 10 minutes.
6. Now push the Temp button and rotate the dial to set the temperature at 355 degrees F.
7. Press "Start/Pause" button to start.
8. When the unit beeps to show that it is preheated, open the lid.
9. Arrange the veggie balls in "Air Fry Basket" and insert in the oven.
10. Serve warm.
- **Nutrition Info:** Calories 43 Total Fat 1.4 g Saturated Fat 0.7 g Cholesterol 3 mg Sodium 155 mg Total Carbs 5.6 g Fiber 1.9 g Sugar 1.2 g Protein 3.1 g

12. Lime Pumpkin Wedges

Servings:4
Cooking Time: 30 Minutes
Ingredients:
- 1 lb pumpkin, cut into wedges
- 1 tbsp paprika
- 1 whole lime, squeezed
- 1 cup paleo dressing
- 1 tbsp balsamic vinegar
- Salt and black pepper to taste
- 1 tsp turmeric

Directions:
1. Preheat Breville on AirFry function to 360 F. Add the pumpkin wedges in a baking tray and press Start. Cook for 20 minutes. In a bowl, mix lime juice, vinegar, turmeric, salt, pepper, and paprika. Pour the mixture over pumpkin and cook for 5 more minutes. Serve.

13. Feta Lime Corn

Servings: 2

Cooking Time: 20 Minutes
Ingredients:
- 2 ears of corn
- Juice of 2 small limes
- 2 tsp paprika
- 4 oz feta cheese, grated

Directions:
1. Preheat Breville Smart on Air Fry function to 370 F. Peel the corn and remove the silk. Place the corn in the baking pan and cook for 15 minutes. Squeeze the juice of 1 lime on top of each ear of corn. Top with feta cheese and serve.

14. Delicious Mac And Cheese

Servings: 6
Cooking Time: 30 Minutes
Ingredients:
- 2 1/2 cups pasta, uncooked
- 1/2 cup cream
- 1 cup vegetable broth
- 2 tbsp flour
- 1/2 cup parmesan cheese, grated
- 1/2 cup Velveeta cheese, cut into small cubes
- 2 cups Colby cheese, shredded
- 2 tbsp butter
- 1 tsp salt

Directions:
1. Fit the Breville Smart oven with the rack in position
2. Cook pasta according to the packet instructions. Drain well.
3. Melt butter in a pan over medium heat. Slowly whisk in flour.
4. Whisk constantly and slowly add the broth.
5. Slowly pour the cream and whisk constantly.
6. Slowly add parmesan cheese, Velveeta cheese, and Colby cheese and whisk until smooth.
7. Add cooked pasta to the sauce and stir well to coat.
8. Transfer pasta into the greased casserole dish.
9. Set to bake at 350 F for 35 minutes. After 5 minutes place the casserole dish in the preheated oven.

10. Serve and enjoy.
- **Nutrition Info:** Calories 410 Fat 21.8 g Carbohydrates 34 g Sugar 1.3 g Protein 20 g Cholesterol 99 mg

15. Baked Asparagus

Servings: 4
Cooking Time: 15 Minutes
Ingredients:
- 30 asparagus spears, cut the ends
- 1/2 tsp garlic powder
- 1 tbsp olive oil
- Pepper
- Salt

Directions:
1. Fit the Breville Smart oven with the rack in position
2. Add asparagus into the large bowl. Drizzle with oil.
3. Sprinkle with garlic powder, pepper, and salt. Toss well.
4. Arrange asparagus in baking pan.
5. Set to bake at 400 F for 20 minutes. After 5 minutes place the baking pan in the preheated oven.
6. Serve and enjoy.
- **Nutrition Info:** Calories 67 Fat 3.7 g Carbohydrates 7.3 g Sugar 3.5 g Protein 4 g Cholesterol 0 mg

16. Creamy Broccoli Casserole

Servings: 6
Cooking Time: 30 Minutes
Ingredients:
- 16 oz frozen broccoli florets, defrosted and drained
- 1/2 tsp onion powder
- 10.5 oz can cream of mushroom soup
- 1 cup cheddar cheese, shredded
- 1/3 cup almond milk
- For topping:
- 1 tbsp butter, melted
- 1/2 cup cracker crumbs

Directions:
1. Fit the Breville Smart oven with the rack in position
2. Add all ingredients except topping ingredients into the 1.5-qt casserole dish.

3. In a small bowl, mix together cracker crumbs and melted butter and sprinkle over the casserole dish mixture.
4. Set to bake at 350 F for 35 minutes. After 5 minutes place the casserole dish in the preheated oven.
5. Serve and enjoy.
- **Nutrition Info:** Calories 203 Fat 13.5 g Carbohydrates 11.9 g Sugar 3.6 g Protein 6.9 g Cholesterol 26 mg

17. Allspice Chicken Wings

Servings: 4
Cooking Time: 45 Minutes
Ingredients:
- ½ tsp celery salt
- ½ tsp bay leaf powder
- ½ tsp ground black pepper
- ½ tsp paprika
- ¼ tsp dry mustard
- ¼ tsp cayenne pepper
- ¼ tsp allspice
- 2 pounds chicken wings

Directions:
1. Preheat your Breville Smart to 340 F on Air Fry function. In a bowl, mix celery salt, bay leaf powder, black pepper, paprika, dry mustard, cayenne pepper, and allspice. Coat the wings thoroughly in this mixture.
2. Arrange the wings in an even layer in the greased frying basket and fit in the baking tray. Cook the chicken until it's no longer pink around the bone, about 20 minutes. Then, increase the temperature to 380 F and cook for 6 minutes more until crispy on the outside. Serve warm.

18. Savory Chicken Nuggets With Parmesan Cheese

Servings: 4
Cooking Time: 25 Minutes
Ingredients:
- 1 lb chicken breasts, cubed
- Salt and black pepper to taste
- 2 tbsp olive oil
- 5 tbsp plain breadcrumbs
- 2 tbsp panko breadcrumbs
- 2 tbsp grated Parmesan cheese

Directions:

1. Preheat Breville Smart on Air Fry function to 380 F. Season the chicken with salt and pepper; set aside. In a bowl, mix the breadcrumbs with the Parmesan cheese.
2. Brush the chicken pieces with the olive oil, then dip into breadcrumb mixture, and transfer to the Air Fryer basket. Fit in the baking tray and lightly spray chicken with cooking spray. Cook for 10 minutes, flipping once halfway through until golden brown on the outside and no more pink on the inside. Serve warm.

19. French-style Fries

Servings: 4
Cooking Time: 35 Minutes
Ingredients:

- 4 russet potatoes, cut into 3-inch pieces
- 2 tbsp olive oil
- Salt and black pepper to taste

Directions:

1. Preheat Breville Smart on Air Fry function to 360 F. Drizzle the potatoes with olive oil and toss to coat. Place the potatoes in the Air Fryer basket and fit in the baking tray. Cook for 20-25 minutes. Sprinkle with salt and pepper and to serve.

20. Ham Rolls With Vegetables & Walnuts

Servings: 4
Cooking Time: 15 Minutes
Ingredients:

- 8 ham slices
- 4 carrots, chopped
- 4 slices ham
- 2 oz walnuts, finely chopped
- 1 zucchini
- 1 clove garlic
- 1 tbsp olive oil
- 1 tbsp ginger powder
- ¼ cup basil leaves, finely chopped
- Salt and black pepper to taste

Directions:

1. Heat the olive oil in a pan over medium heat and add the zucchini, carrots, garlic, ginger and salt; cook for 5 minutes. Add the basil and walnuts, and keep stirring.
2. Divide the mixture between the ham slices. Then fold one side above the filling and roll in. Cook the rolls in the preheated Breville Smart for 8 minutes at 300 F on Bake function.

21. Mini Salmon & Cheese Quiches

Servings:15
Cooking Time: 20 Minutes
Ingredients:

- 15 mini tart cases
- 4 eggs, lightly beaten
- ½ cup heavy cream
- Salt and black pepper
- 3 oz smoked salmon
- 6 oz cream cheese, divided into 15 pieces
- 6 fresh dill

Directions:

1. Mix together eggs and heavy cream in a pourable measuring container. Arrange the tarts on the basket. Fill them with the mixture, halfway up the side and top with salmon and cream cheese. Bake for 10 minutes at 340 F on Bake function, regularly checking to avoid overcooking. Sprinkle with dill and serve chilled.

22. Cinnamon-spiced Acorn Squash

Servings:2
Cooking Time: 15 Minutes
Ingredients:

- 1 medium acorn squash, halved crosswise and deseeded
- 1 teaspoon coconut oil
- 1 teaspoon light brown sugar
- Few dashes of ground cinnamon
- Few dashes of ground nutmeg

Directions:

1. On a clean work surface, rub the cut sides of the acorn squash with coconut oil. Scatter with the brown sugar, cinnamon, and nutmeg.
2. Put the squash halves in the air fryer basket, cut-side up.
3. Put the air fryer basket on the baking pan and slide into Rack Position 2, select Air Fry, set temperature to 325ºF (163ºC), and set time to 15 minutes.

4. When cooking is complete, the squash halves should be just tender when pierced in the center with a paring knife. Remove from the oven. Rest for 5 to 10 minutes and serve warm.
5. Parmesan Asparagus Fries
6. Prep time: 15 minutes | Cooking time: 6 minutes | Servings:4
7. egg whites
8. ¼ cup water
9. ¼ cup plus 2 tablespoons grated Parmesan cheese, divided
10. ¾ cup panko bread crumbs
11. ¼ teaspoon salt
12. ounces (340 g) fresh asparagus spears, woody ends trimmed
13. Cooking spray
14. In a shallow dish, whisk together the egg whites and water until slightly foamy. In a separate shallow dish, thoroughly combine ¼ cup of Parmesan cheese, bread crumbs, and salt.
15. Dip the asparagus in the egg white, then roll in the cheese mixture to coat well.
16. Place the asparagus in the air fryer basket in a single layer, leaving space between each spear. Spritz the asparagus with cooking spray.
17. Put the air fryer basket on the baking pan and slide into Rack Position 2, select Air Fry, set temperature to 390ºF (199ºC), and set time to 6 minutes.
18. When cooking is complete, the asparagus should be golden brown and crisp. Remove from the oven. Sprinkle with the remaining 2 tablespoons of cheese and serve hot.

23. Wonton Poppers

Servings: 10
Cooking Time: 10 Minutes
Ingredients:
- Nonstick cooking spray
- 1 package refrigerated square wonton wrappers
- 1 8-ounce package cream cheese, softened
- 3 jalapenos, seeds and ribs removed, finely chopped
- 1/2 cup shredded cheddar cheese

Directions:
1. Place baking pan in position 2 of the oven. Lightly spray fryer basket with cooking spray.
2. In a large bowl, combine all ingredients except the wrappers until combined.
3. Lay wrappers in a single layer on a baking sheet. Spoon a teaspoon of filling in the center. Moisten the edges with water and fold wrappers over filling, pinching edges to seal. Place in a single layer in the basket.
4. Place the basket in the oven and set to air fry on 375°F for 10 minutes. Cook until golden brown and crisp, turning over halfway through cooking time. Repeat with remaining ingredients. Serve immediately.
- **Nutrition Info:** Calories 287, Total Fat 11g, Saturated Fat 6g, Total Carbs 38g, Net Carbs 37g, Protein 9g, Sugar 1g, Fiber 1g, Sodium 485mg, Potassium 98mg, Phosphorus 104mg

24. Chickpeas With Rosemary & Sage

Servings: 4
Cooking Time: 20 Minutes
Ingredients:
- 2 (14.5-ounce) cans chickpeas, rinsed
- 2 tbsp olive oil
- 1 tsp dried rosemary
- ½ tsp dried thyme
- ¼ tsp dried sage
- ¼ tsp salt

Directions:
1. In a bowl, mix together chickpeas, oil, rosemary, thyme, sage, and salt. Transfer them to the Breville Smart Air Fryer baking dish and spread in an even layer. Cook for 15 minutes at 380 F on Bake function, shaking once halfway through cooking. Serve.

25. Rosemary Potatoes

Servings:4
Cooking Time: 35 Minutes
Ingredients:
- 1 ½ pounds potatoes, halved
- 2 tbsp olive oil
- 3 garlic cloves, minced

- 1 tbsp minced fresh rosemary
- Salt and black pepper to taste

Directions:

1. In a bowl, mix potatoes, olive oil, garlic, rosemary, salt, and pepper. Arrange the potatoes on the basket. Select AirFry function, adjust the temperature to 380 F, and press Start. Cook for 20-25 minutes until crispy on the outside and tender on the inside. Serve warm.

26. Puffed Asparagus Spears

Servings: 10
Cooking Time: 10 Minutes
Ingredients:

- Nonstick cooking spray
- 3 oz. prosciutto, sliced thin & cut in 30 long strips
- 30 asparagus spears, trimmed
- 10 (14 x 9-inch) sheets phyllo dough, thawed

Directions:

1. Place baking pan in position 2 of the oven.
2. Wrap each asparagus spear with a piece of prosciutto, like a barber pole.
3. One at a time, place a sheet of phyllo on a work surface and cut into 3 4 1/2x9-inch rectangles.
4. Place an asparagus spear across a short end and roll up. Place in a single layer in the fryer basket. Spray with cooking spray.
5. Place the basket in the oven and set to air fry on 450°F for 10 minutes. Cook until phyllo is crisp and golden, about 8-10 minutes, turning over halfway through cooking time. Repeat with remaining ingredients. Serve warm.
- **Nutrition Info:** Calories 74, Total Fat 2g, Saturated Fat 0g, Total Carbs 11g, Net Carbs 10g, Protein 3g, Sugar 0g, Fiber 1g, Sodium 189mg, Potassium 60mg, Phosphorus 33mg

27. Goat Cheese & Pancetta Bombs

Servings: 10
Cooking Time: 25 Minutes
Ingredients:

- 16 oz soft goat cheese
- 2 tbsp fresh rosemary, finely chopped
- 1 cup almonds, chopped into small pieces
- Salt and black pepper
- 15 dried plums, chopped
- 15 pancetta slices

Directions:

1. Line the Breville Smart Air Fryer tray with parchment paper. In a bowl, add goat cheese, rosemary, almonds, salt, pepper, and plums; stir well. Roll into balls and wrap with pancetta slices. Arrange the bombs on the tray and cook for 10 minutes at 400 F. Let cool before serving.

28. Vegetable And Egg Salad

Servings: 4
Cooking Time: 20 Minutes
Ingredients:

- 1/3-pound Brussels sprouts
- 1/2 cup radishes, sliced
- 1/2 cup mozzarella cheese, crumbled
- 1 red onion, chopped
- 4 eggs, hardboiled and sliced
- Dressing:
- 1/4 cup olive oil
- 2 tablespoons champagne vinegar
- 1 teaspoon Dijon mustard
- Sea salt and ground black pepper, to taste

Directions:

1. Start by preheating your Air Fryer to 380 degrees F.
2. Add the Brussels sprouts andradishes to the cooking basket. Spritz with cooking spray and cook for 15 minutes. Let it cool to room temperature about 15 minutes.
3. Toss the vegetables with cheese and red onion.
4. Mix all ingredients for the dressing and toss to combine well. Serve topped with the hardboiled eggs.
- **Nutrition Info:** 298 Calories; 23g Fat; 5g Carbs; 15g Protein; 6g Sugars; 6g FiberSimple Stuffed Bell Peppers

29. Easy Home Fries(1)

Servings: 4
Cooking Time: 20 Minutes
Ingredients:

- ½ medium white onion; peeled and diced

- 1 medium green bell pepper; seeded and diced
- 1 medium jicama; peeled.
- 1 tbsp. coconut oil; melted
- ½ tsp. pink Himalayan salt
- ¼ tsp. ground black pepper

Directions:

1. Cut jicama into 1-inch cubes. Place into a large bowl and toss with coconut oil until coated. Sprinkle with pepper and salt. Place into the air fryer basket with peppers and onion.
2. Adjust the temperature to 400 Degrees F and set the timer for 10 minutes. Shake two or three times during cooking. Jicama will be tender and dark around edges. Serve immediately.

- **Nutrition Info:** Calories: 97; Protein: 5g; Fiber: 0g; Fat: 3g; Carbs: 18g

30. Garlic Lemon Roasted Chicken

Servings: 4
Cooking Time: 60 Minutes
Ingredients:

- 1 (3 ½ pounds) whole chicken
- 2 tbsp olive oil
- Salt and black pepper to taste
- 1 lemon, cut into quarters
- 5 garlic cloves

Directions:

1. Preheat Breville Smart on Air Fry function to 360 F. Brush the chicken with olive oil and season with salt and pepper. Stuff with lemon and garlic cloves into the cavity.
2. Place the chicken breast-side down onto the Breville Smart Air Fryer basket. Tuck the legs and wings tips under. Fit in the baking tray and cook for 45 minutes at 350 F on Bake function. Let rest for 5-6 minutes, then carve and serve.

31. Sesame Cabbage & Prawn Egg Roll Wraps

Servings:4
Cooking Time: 25 Minutes
Ingredients:

- 2 tbsp vegetable oil
- 1-inch piece fresh ginger, grated
- 1 tbsp minced garlic
- 1 carrot, cut into strips

- ¼ cup chicken broth
- 2 tbsp soy sauce
- 1 tbsp sugar
- 1 cup shredded Napa cabbage
- 1 tbsp sesame oil
- 8 cooked prawns, minced
- 1 egg
- 8 egg roll wrappers

Directions:

1. Warm vegetable oil In a skillet over high heat and sauté ginger and garlic for 40 seconds until fragrant. Stir in carrot and cook for another 2 minutes. Pour in chicken broth, soy sauce, and sugar and bring to a boil. Add cabbage and let simmer until softened, for 4 minutes.
2. Remove the skillet from the heat and stir in sesame oil. Strain cabbage mixture and fold in minced prawns. Whisk an egg in a small bowl. Fill each egg roll wrapper with prawn mixture, arranging the mixture just below the center of the wrapper.
3. Fold the bottom part over the filling and tuck under. Fold in both sides and tightly roll up. Use the whisked egg to seal the wrapper. Place the rolls into the frying basket and spray with oil. Select AirFry function, adjust the temperature to 380 F, and press Start. Cook for 12 minutes.

32. Baked Cauliflower & Tomatoes

Servings: 4
Cooking Time: 20 Minutes
Ingredients:

- 4 cups cauliflower florets
- 1 tbsp capers, drained
- 3 tbsp olive oil
- 1/2 cup cherry tomatoes, halved
- 2 tbsp fresh parsley, chopped
- 2 garlic cloves, sliced
- Pepper
- Salt

Directions:

1. Fit the Breville Smart oven with the rack in position
2. In a bowl, toss together cherry tomatoes, cauliflower, oil, garlic, capers, pepper, and salt and spread in baking pan.
3. Set to bake at 450 F for 25 minutes. After 5 minutes place the baking pan in the preheated oven.

4. Garnish with parsley and serve.
- **Nutrition Info:** Calories 123 Fat 10.7 g Carbohydrates 6.9 g Sugar 3 g Protein 2.4 g Cholesterol 0 mg

33. Roasted Garlic(1)

Servings: 12 Cloves
Cooking Time: 20 Minutes
Ingredients:
- 1 medium head garlic
- 2 tsp. avocado oil

Directions:
1. Remove any hanging excess peel from the garlic but leave the cloves covered. Cut off ¼ of the head of garlic, exposing the tips of the cloves
2. Drizzle with avocado oil. Place the garlic head into a small sheet of aluminum foil, completely enclosing it. Place it into the air fryer basket. Adjust the temperature to 400 Degrees F and set the timer for 20 minutes. If your garlic head is a bit smaller, check it after 15 minutes
3. When done, garlic should be golden brown and very soft
4. To serve, cloves should pop out and easily be spread or sliced. Store in an airtight container in the refrigerator up to 5 days.
5. You may also freeze individual cloves on a baking sheet, then store together in a freezer-safe storage bag once frozen.
- **Nutrition Info:** Calories: 11; Protein: 0.2g; Fiber: 0.1g; Fat: 0.7g; Carbs: 1.0g

34. Maple Shrimp With Coconut

Servings: 3
Cooking Time: 30 Minutes
Ingredients:
- 1 lb jumbo shrimp, peeled and deveined
- ¾ cup shredded coconut
- 1 tbsp maple syrup
- ½ cup breadcrumbs
- ⅓ cup cornstarch
- ½ cup milk

Directions:
1. Pour the cornstarch in a zipper bag, add shrimp, zip the bag up and shake vigorously to coat with the cornstarch. Mix the syrup and milk in a bowl and set aside.
2. In a separate bowl, mix the breadcrumbs and shredded coconut. Open the zipper bag and remove each shrimp while shaking off excess starch. Dip shrimp in the milk mixture and then in the crumb mixture while pressing loosely to trap enough crumbs and coconut.
3. Place in the basket without overcrowding and fit in the baking tray. Cook for 12 minutes at 350 F on Air Fry function, flipping once halfway through until golden brown. Serve warm.

35. Creamy Corn Casserole

Servings:4
Cooking Time: 15 Minutes
Ingredients:
- 2 cups frozen yellow corn
- 1 egg, beaten
- 3 tablespoons flour
- ½ cup grated Swiss or Havarti cheese
- ½ cup light cream
- ¼ cup milk
- Pinch salt
- Freshly ground black pepper, to taste
- 2 tablespoons butter, cut into cubes
- Nonstick cooking spray

Directions:
1. Spritz the baking pan with nonstick cooking spray.
2. Stir together the remaining ingredients except the butter in a medium bowl until well incorporated. Transfer the mixture to the prepared baking pan and scatter with the butter cubes.
3. Slide the baking pan into Rack Position 1, select Convection Bake, set temperature to 320ºF (160ºC), and set time to 15 minutes.
4. When cooking is complete, the top should be golden brown and a toothpick inserted in the center should come out clean. Remove from the oven. Let the casserole cool for 5 minutes before slicing into wedges and serving.

36. Sausage Mushroom Caps(1)

Servings: 2
Cooking Time: 20 Minutes
Ingredients:
- ½ lb. Italian sausage
- 6 large Portobello mushroom caps
- ¼ cup grated Parmesan cheese.
- ¼ cup chopped onion

- 2 tbsp. blanched finely ground almond flour
- 1 tsp. minced fresh garlic

Directions:
1. Use a spoon to hollow out each mushroom cap, reserving scrapings.
2. In a medium skillet over medium heat, brown the sausage about 10 minutes or until fully cooked and no pink remains. Drain and then add reserved mushroom scrapings, onion, almond flour, Parmesan and garlic.
3. Gently fold ingredients together and continue cooking an additional minute, then remove from heat
4. Evenly spoon the mixture into mushroom caps and place the caps into a 6-inch round pan. Place pan into the air fryer basket
5. Adjust the temperature to 375 Degrees F and set the timer for 8 minutes. When finished cooking, the tops will be browned and bubbling. Serve warm.
- **Nutrition Info:** Calories: 404; Protein: 23g; Fiber: 5g; Fat: 28g; Carbs: 12g

37. Holiday Pumpkin Wedges

Servings: 3
Cooking Time: 30 Minutes
Ingredients:
- ½ pumpkin, washed and cut into wedges
- 1 tbsp paprika
- 1 whole lime, squeezed
- 1 cup paleo dressing
- 1 tbsp balsamic vinegar
- Salt and black pepper to taste
- 1 tsp turmeric

Directions:
1. Preheat Breville Smart on Air Fry function to 360 F. Place the pumpkin wedges in your Air Fryer baking tray and cook for 20 minutes. In a bowl, mix lime juice, vinegar, turmeric, salt, pepper and paprika to form a marinade. Pour the marinade over pumpkin and cook for 5 more minutes.

38. Garlic Potato Chips

Servings: 3
Cooking Time: 30 Minutes + Marinating Time
Ingredients:
- 3 whole potatoes, cut into thin slices
- ¼ cup olive oil
- 1 tbsp garlic
- ½ cup cream
- 2 tbsp rosemary

Directions:
1. Preheat Breville Smart on Air Fry function to 390 F. In a bowl, add oil, garlic, and salt to form a marinade. Stir in the potatoes. Allow sitting for 30 minutes.
2. Lay the potato slices onto the Air Fryer basket and fit in the baking tray. Cook for 20 minutes. After 10 minutes, give the chips a turn. When readt, sprinkle with rosemary and serve.

39. Baked Broccoli

Servings: 6
Cooking Time: 20 Minutes
Ingredients:
- 4 cups broccoli florets
- 3 tbsp olive oil
- 1/2 tsp pepper
- 1/2 tsp garlic powder
- 1 tsp Italian seasoning
- 1 tsp salt

Directions:
1. Fit the Breville Smart oven with the rack in position
2. Spread broccoli in baking pan and drizzle with oil and season with garlic powder, Italian seasoning, pepper, and salt.
3. Set to bake at 400 F for 25 minutes. After 5 minutes place the baking pan in the preheated oven.
4. Serve and enjoy.
- **Nutrition Info:** Calories 84 Fat 7.4 g Carbohydrates 4.4 g Sugar 1.2 g Protein 1.8 g Cholesterol 1 mg

BREAKFAST RECIPES

40. Classic Bacon & Egg English Muffin

Servings: 1
Cooking Time: 15 Minutes
Ingredients:
- 1 egg
- 1 English muffin
- 2 slices of bacon
- Salt and black pepper to taste

Directions:
1. Preheat Breville Smart on Bake function to 395 F. Crack the egg into a ramekin. Place the English muffin, egg ramekin, and bacon in a baking pan. Cook for 9 minutes. Let cool slightly so you can assemble the sandwich. Cut the muffin in half. Place the egg on one half and season with salt and pepper. Arrange the bacon on top. Top with the other muffin half.

41. Air Fried Philly Cheesesteaks

Servings:2
Cooking Time: 20 Minutes
Ingredients:
- 12 ounces (340 g) boneless rib-eye steak, sliced thinly
- ½ teaspoon Worcestershire sauce
- ½ teaspoon soy sauce
- Kosher salt and ground black pepper, to taste
- ½ green bell pepper, stemmed, deseeded, and thinly sliced
- ½ small onion, halved and thinly sliced
- 1 tablespoon vegetable oil
- 2 soft hoagie rolls, split three-fourths of the way through
- 1 tablespoon butter, softened
- 2 slices provolone cheese, halved

Directions:
1. Combine the steak, Worcestershire sauce, soy sauce, salt, and ground black pepper in a large bowl. Toss to coat well. Set aside.
2. Combine the bell pepper, onion, salt, ground black pepper, and vegetable oil in a separate bowl. Toss to coat the vegetables well.
3. Place the steak and vegetables in the air fryer basket.
4. Put the air fryer basket on the baking pan and slide into Rack Position 2, select Air Fry, set temperature to 400ºF (205ºC) and set time to 15 minutes.
5. When cooked, the steak will be browned and vegetables will be tender. Transfer them onto a plate. Set aside.
6. Brush the hoagie rolls with butter and place in the basket.
7. Select Toast and set time to 3 minutes. Return to the oven. When done, the rolls should be lightly browned.
8. Transfer the rolls to a clean work surface and divide the steak and vegetable mix between the rolls. Spread with cheese. Transfer the stuffed rolls to the basket.
9. Select Air Fry and set time to 2 minutes. Return to the oven. When done, the cheese should be melted.
10. Serve immediately.

42. Spinach Egg Breakfast

Servings: 4
Cooking Time: 20 Minutes
Ingredients:
- 3 eggs
- 1/4 cup coconut milk
- 1/4 cup parmesan cheese, grated 4 oz spinach, chopped
- 3 oz cottage cheese

Directions:
1. Preheat the air fryer to 350 F.
2. Add eggs, milk, half parmesan cheese, and cottage cheese in a bowl and whisk well. Add spinach and stir well.
3. Pour mixture into the air fryer baking dish.
4. Sprinkle remaining half parmesan cheese on top.
5. Place dish in the air fryer and cook for 20 minutes.
6. Serve and enjoy.
- **Nutrition Info:** Calories 144 Fat 8.5 g Carbohydrates 2.5 g Sugar 1.1 g Protein 14 g Cholesterol 135 mg

43. Baked Eggs

Servings: 4
Cooking Time: 15-20 | Minutes
Ingredients:

- 7 Oz. leg ham
- 4 eggs
- 4 tsps full cream milk Margarine
- 1 lb baby spinach
- 1 tablespoon olive oil Salt and Pepper to taste

Directions:

1. Preheat the Air Fryer to 350°F. Layer four ramekins with margarine.
2. Equally divide the spinach and ham into the four ramekins. Break 1 egg into each and add a tsp. of milk. Spice with salt and pepper.
3. Place into Air Fryer for about 15-20 minutes. For a runny yolk, cook for 15 minutes, for fully cooked; 20 minutes.
- **Nutrition Info:** Calories 113 Fat 8.2 g Carbohydrates 0.3 g Sugar 0.2 g Protein 5.4 g Cholesterol 18 mg

44. Peanut Butter And Jelly Banana Boats

Servings: 1
Cooking Time: 15 Minutes
Ingredients:

- 1 banana
- 1/4 cup peanut butter
- 1/4 cup jelly
- 1 tablespoon granola

Directions:

1. Start by preheating toaster oven to 350°F.
2. Slice banana lengthwise and separate slightly.
3. Spread peanut butter and jelly in the gap.
4. Sprinkle granola over the entire banana.
5. Bake for 15 minutes.
- **Nutrition Info:** Calories: 724, Sodium: 327 mg, Dietary Fiber: 9.2 g, Total Fat: 36.6 g, Total Carbs: 102.9 g, Protein: 20.0 g.

45. Vanilla Raspberry Pancakes With Maple Syrup

Servings:4
Cooking Time: 15 Minutes
Ingredients:

- 2 cups all-purpose flour
- 1 cup milk
- 3 eggs, beaten
- 1 tsp baking powder
- 1 cup brown sugar
- 1 ½ tsp vanilla extract
- ½ cup frozen raspberries, thawed
- 2 tbsp maple syrup
- A pinch of salt

Directions:

1. Preheat Breville on Bake function to 390 F. In a bowl, mix flour, baking powder, salt, milk, eggs, vanilla extract, sugar, and maple syrup until smooth. Stir in the raspberries.
2. Drop the batter onto a greased baking dish. Just make sure to leave some space between the pancakes. Press Start and cook for 10 minutes. Serve.

46. Tator Tots Casserole

Servings: 8
Cooking Time: 30 Minutes
Ingredients:

- 8 eggs
- 28 oz tator tots
- 8 oz pepper jack cheese, shredded
- 2 green onions, sliced
- 1/4 cup milk
- 1 lb breakfast sausage, cooked
- Pepper
- Salt

Directions:

1. Fit the Breville Smart oven with the rack in position
2. Spray 13*9-inch baking pan with cooking spray and set aside.
3. In a bowl, whisk eggs with milk, pepper, and salt.
4. Layer sausage in a prepared baking pan then pour the egg mixture and sprinkle with half shredded cheese and green onions.
5. Add tator tots on top.
6. Set to bake at 400 F for 35 minutes. After 5 minutes place the baking pan in the preheated oven.
7. Top with remaining cheese and serve.

- **Nutrition Info:** Calories 398 Fat 31.5 g Carbohydrates 2 g Sugar 0.8 g Protein 22.1 g Cholesterol 251 mg

47. Olives And Kale

Servings: 4
Cooking Time: 30 Minutes
Ingredients:
- 4 eggs; whisked
- 1 cup kale; chopped.
- ½ cup black olives, pitted and sliced
- 2 tbsp. cheddar; grated
- Cooking spray
- A pinch of salt and black pepper

Directions:
1. Take a bowl and mix the eggs with the rest of the ingredients except the cooking spray and whisk well.
2. Now, take a pan that fits in your air fryer and grease it with the cooking spray, pour the olives mixture inside, spread
3. Put the pan into the machine and cook at 360°F for 20 minutes. Serve for breakfast hot.
- **Nutrition Info:** Calories: 220; Fat: 13g; Fiber: 4g; Carbs: 6g; Protein: 12g

48. Caprese Sourdough Sandwich

Servings:2
Cooking Time: 25 Minutes
Ingredients:
- 4 sourdough bread slices
- 2 tbsp mayonnaise
- 2 slices ham
- 2 lettuce leaves
- 1 tomato, sliced
- 2 mozzarella cheese slices
- Salt and black pepper to taste

Directions:
1. On a clean board, lay the sourdough slices and spread with mayonnaise. Top 2 of the slices with ham, lettuce, tomato and mozzarella. Season with salt and pepper. Top with the remaining two slices to form two sandwiches. Spray with oil and transfer to the frying basket. Cook in the preheated Breville oven for 14 minutes at 340 F on Bake function.

49. Egg In A Hole

Servings:1
Cooking Time: 5 Minutes
Ingredients:
- 1 slice bread
- 1 teaspoon butter, softened
- 1 egg
- Salt and pepper, to taste
- 1 tablespoon shredded Cheddar cheese
- 2 teaspoons diced ham

Directions:
1. On a flat work surface, cut a hole in the center of the bread slice with a 2½-inch-diameter biscuit cutter.
2. Spread the butter evenly on each side of the bread slice and transfer to the baking pan.
3. Crack the egg into the hole and season as desired with salt and pepper. Scatter the shredded cheese and diced ham on top.
4. Slide the baking pan into Rack Position 1, select Convection Bake, set temperature to 330ºF (166ºC), and set time to 5 minutes.
5. When cooking is complete, the bread should be lightly browned and the egg should be set. Remove from the oven and serve hot.

50. Pancetta & Hot Dogs Omelet

Servings: 2
Cooking Time: 10 Minutes
Ingredients:
- 4 eggs
- ¼ teaspoon dried parsley
- ¼ teaspoon dried rosemary
- 1 pancetta slice, chopped
- 2 hot dogs, chopped
- 2 small onions, chopped

Directions:
1. In a bowl, crack the eggs and beat well.
2. Add the remaining ingredients and gently, stir to combine.
3. Place the mixture into a baking pan.
4. Press "Power Button" of Air Fry Oven and turn the dial to select the "Air Fry" mode.
5. Press the Time button and again turn the dial to set the cooking time to 10 minutes.
6. Now push the Temp button and rotate the dial to set the temperature at 320 degrees F.
7. Press "Start/Pause" button to start.

8. When the unit beeps to show that it is preheated, open the lid.
9. Arrange pan over the "Wire Rack" and insert in the oven.
10. Cut into equal-sized wedges and serve hot.
- **Nutrition Info:** Calories 282 Total Fat 19.3 g Saturated Fat 6.5 g Cholesterol 351mg Sodium 632 mg Total Carbs 8.2 g Fiber 1.6 g Sugar 4.2 g Protein 18.9 g

51. Chives Salmon And Shrimp Bowls

Servings: 4
Cooking Time: 12 Minutes
Ingredients:
- 1 pound shrimp, peeled and deveined
- ½ pound salmon fillets, boneless and cubed
- 2 spring onions, chopped
- 2 teaspoons olive oil
- 1 cup baby kale
- Salt and black pepper to the taste
- 1 tablespoon chives, chopped

Directions:
1. Preheat the air fryer with the oil at 330 degrees F, add the shrimp, salmon and the other ingredients, toss gently and cook for 12 minutes.
2. Divide everything into bowls and serve.
- **Nutrition Info:** calories 244, fat 11, fiber 4, carbs 5, protein 7

52. Simple Apple Crisp

Servings: 8
Cooking Time: 35 Minutes
Ingredients:
- 4 medium apples, peel & slice
- 1 tsp cinnamon
- 4 tbsp sugar
- For topping:
- 1/3 cup butter, melted
- 1/2 cup brown sugar
- 3/4 cup all-purpose flour
- 3/4 cup rolled oats

Directions:
1. Fit the Breville Smart oven with the rack in position
2. Add sliced apples, cinnamon, and sugar in a greased 9-inch baking dish and mix well.

3. In a bowl, mix oats, brown sugar, and flour. Add melted butter and mix well.
4. Sprinkle oat mixture over sliced apples.
5. Set to bake at 375 F for 40 minutes. After 5 minutes place the baking dish in the preheated oven.
6. Serve and enjoy.
- **Nutrition Info:** Calories 255 Fat 8.5 g Carbohydrates 44.7 g Sugar 26.5 g Protein 2.6 g Cholesterol 20 mg

53. Soft Banana Oat Muffins

Servings: 12
Cooking Time: 20 Minutes
Ingredients:
- 1 egg
- 1 cup banana, mashed
- 1 tsp vanilla
- 1/3 cup applesauce
- 3/4 cup milk
- 1/4 tsp nutmeg
- 1/2 tsp cinnamon
- 1 tsp baking soda
- 2 tsp baking powder
- 1/4 cup brown sugar
- 1/4 cup white sugar
- 1 cup old fashioned oats
- 1 1/2 cups whole wheat flour
- 1/2 tsp salt

Directions:
1. Fit the Breville Smart oven with the rack in position
2. Line a 12-cup muffin tray with cupcake liners and set aside.
3. In a mixing bowl, mix flour, nutmeg, cinnamon, baking soda, baking powder, sugar, oats, flour, and salt.
4. In a separate bowl, whisk eggs with milk, vanilla, and applesauce. Add mashed banana and stir to combine.
5. Add flour mixture into the egg mixture and mix until just combined.
6. Pour mixture into the prepared muffin tray.
7. Set to bake at 400 F for 25 minutes. After 5 minutes place the muffin tray in the preheated oven.
8. Serve and enjoy.

- **Nutrition Info:** Calories 165 Fat 1.7 g Carbohydrates 33 g Sugar 10.5 g Protein 4.4 g Cholesterol 15 mg

54. Brioche Breakfast Pudding

Servings: 8
Cooking Time: 45 Minutes
Ingredients:

- 1 loaf brioche bread, cut in cubes
- ½ tbsp. coconut oil, soft
- 4 cups milk
- 1 can coconut milk
- 6 eggs
- ½ cup sugar
- 2 tsp vanilla
- ¼ tsp salt
- 1 cup coconut, shredded
- ½ cup chocolate chips

Directions:

1. Place rack in position 1 of the oven. Grease an 8x11-inch baking pan with coconut oil.
2. Add the bread cubes to the pan, pressing lightly to settle.
3. In a large bowl, whisk together milk, coconut milk, eggs, sugar, vanilla, and salt until combined.
4. Stir in coconut and chocolate chips. Pour evenly over bread. Cover with plastic wrap and refrigerate 2 hours or overnight.
5. Set oven to bake on 350°F for 50 minutes. After 5 minutes, add the pudding to the oven and bake 40-45 minutes, or until top is beginning to brown and it passes the toothpick test.
6. Remove to wire rack and let cool 5-10 minutes before serving.
- **Nutrition Info:** Calories 476, Total Fat 24g, Saturated Fat 15g, Total Carbs 51g, Net Carbs 48g, Protein 14g, Sugar 30g, Fiber 3g, Sodium 398mg, Potassium 443mg, Phosphorus 288mg

55. Coconut Brown Rice Porridge With Dates

Servings:1 Or 2
Cooking Time: 23 Minutes
Ingredients:

- ½ cup cooked brown rice
- 1 cup canned coconut milk
- ¼ cup unsweetened shredded coconut
- ¼ cup packed dark brown sugar
- 4 large Medjool dates, pitted and roughly chopped
- ½ teaspoon kosher salt
- ¼ teaspoon ground cardamom
- Heavy cream, for serving (optional)

Directions:

1. Place all the ingredients except the heavy cream in the baking pan and stir until blended.
2. Slide the baking pan into Rack Position 1, select Convection Bake, set temperature to 375ºF (190ºC) and set time to 23 minutes.
3. Stir the porridge halfway through the cooking time.
4. When cooked, the porridge will be thick and creamy.
5. Remove from the oven and ladle the porridge into bowls.
6. Serve hot with a drizzle of the cream, if desired.

56. Cinnamon Sweet Potato Chips

Servings: 6 To 8 Slices
Cooking Time: 8 Minutes
Ingredients:

- 1 small sweet potato, cut into ⅜ inch-thick slices
- 2 tablespoons olive oil
- 1 to 2 teaspoon ground cinnamon

Directions:

1. Add the sweet potato slices and olive oil in a bowl and toss to coat. Fold in the cinnamon and stir to combine.
2. Lay the sweet potato slices in a single layer in the air fryer basket.
3. Put the air fryer basket on the baking pan and slide into Rack Position 2, select Air Fry, set temperature to 390ºF (199ºC), and set time to 8 minutes.
4. Stir the potato slices halfway through the cooking time.
5. When cooking is complete, the chips should be crisp. Remove the pan from the oven. Allow to cool for 5 minutes before serving.

57. Yogurt & Cream Cheese Zucchini Cakes

Servings: 4
Cooking Time: 20 Minutes
Ingredients:

- 1 ½ cups flour
- 1 tsp cinnamon
- 3 eggs
- 2 tsp baking powder
- 2 tbsp sugar
- 1 cup milk
- 2 tbsp butter, melted
- 1 tbsp yogurt
- ½ cup shredded zucchini
- 2 tbsp cream cheese

Directions:

1. In a bowl, whisk the eggs along with the sugar, salt, cinnamon, cream cheese, flour, and baking powder. In another bowl, combine all of the liquid ingredients. Gently combine the dry and liquid mixtures. Stir in zucchini.
2. Line muffin tins with baking paper, and pour the batter inside them. Arrange on the Air Fryer tray and cook for 15-18 minutes on Bake function at 380 F. Serve chilled.

58. Peppery Sausage & Parsley Patties

Servings: 4
Cooking Time: 20 Minutes
Ingredients:

- 1 lb ground Italian sausage
- ¼ cup breadcrumbs
- 1 tsp dried parsley
- 1 tsp red pepper flakes
- ½ tsp salt
- ¼ tsp black pepper
- ¼ tsp garlic powder
- 1 egg, beaten

Directions:

1. Preheat Breville Smart on Bake function to 350 F. Combine all of the ingredients in a large bowl. Line a baking sheet with parchment paper. Make patties out of the sausage mixture and arrange them on the baking sheet. Cook for 15 minutes, flipping once halfway through cooking. Serve.

59. Zucchini Squash Pita Sandwiches Recipe

Servings:x
Cooking Time:x
Ingredients:

- 1 small Zucchini Squash, (5-6 ounces)
- Salt and Pepper, to taste
- 2 Whole Wheat Pitas
- 1/2 cup Hummus
- 1 1/2 cups Fresh Spinach, (2 handfuls)
- 1/2 cup Diced Red Bell Pepper, (about half a large pepper)
- 1/2 cup Chopped Red Onion, (about 1/4 a large onion)
- 2 teaspoons Olive Oil
- 1/4 teaspoon Dried Oregano
- 1/4 teaspoon Dried Thyme
- 1/4 teaspoon Garlic Powder
- 2 tablespoons Crumbled Feta Cheese, (about 1 ounce)

Directions:

1. Adjust the cooking rack to the lowest placement and preheat toaster oven to 425°F on the BAKE setting.
2. While the oven preheats, quarter the zucchini lengthwise and then cut into 1/2-inch thick pieces. Cut the bell pepper and onion into 1-inch thick pieces.
3. Add the vegetables to a roasting pan. Drizzle with oil and sprinkle over the oregano, garlic powder, and salt and pepper, to taste. Toss to combine.
4. Roast vegetables for 10 minutes. Carefully remove the pan and stir. Return pan to oven and continue cooking until the vegetables have softened and started to brown, about 5 minutes more. Remove from the toaster oven and set aside.
5. Reduce the temperature to 375°F and warm the pitas by placing them directly on the cooking rack for 1 to 2 minutes.
6. Spread warm pitas with hummus. Layer with spinach, roasted vegetables, and crumbled feta.

60. Creamy Parmesan & Ham Shirred Eggs

Servings: 2
Cooking Time: 20 Minutes
Ingredients:
- 2 tsp butter
- 4 eggs, divided
- 2 tbsp heavy cream
- 4 slices of ham
- 3 tbsp Parmesan cheese, shredded
- ¼ tsp paprika
- ¾ tsp salt
- ¼ tsp pepper
- 2 tsp chopped chives

Directions:
1. Preheat Breville Smart on Bake function to 320 F. Grease a pie pan with the butter. Arrange the ham slices on the bottom of the pan to cover it completely. Whisk one egg along with the heavy cream, salt, and pepper in a bowl.
2. Pour the mixture over the ham slices. Crack the other eggs over the ham. Sprinkle with Parmesan cheese. Cook for 14 minutes. Season with paprika, garnish with chives, and serve.

61. Zucchini Fritters

Servings: 4
Cooking Time: 7 Minutes
Ingredients:
- 10½ ounces zucchini, grated and squeezed
- 7 ounces Halloumi cheese
- ¼ cup all-purpose flour
- 2 eggs
- 1 teaspoon fresh dill, minced
- Salt and black pepper, to taste

Directions:
1. Preheat the Air fryer to 360 ºF and grease a baking dish.
2. Mix together all the ingredients in a large bowl.
3. Make small fritters from this mixture and place them on the prepared baking dish.
4. Transfer the dish in the Air Fryer basket and cook for about 7 minutes.
5. Dish out and serve warm.

- **Nutrition Info:** Calories: 250 Cal Total Fat: 17.2 g Saturated Fat: 0 g Cholesterol: 0 mg Sodium: 330 mg Total Carbs: 10 g Fiber: 0 g Sugar: 2.7 g Protein: 15.2 g

62. Grilled Cheese Sandwich

Servings: 1 Person
Cooking Time: 12 Minutes
Ingredients:
- 2 slices of bread
- 2 pieces of bacon
- ½ tsp of olive oil side
- Tomatoes
- Jack cheese
- Peach preserves

Directions:
1. If you have left over bacon from air fried bacon recipe you can get two pieces. However, if you do not have any leftover bacon you can get two pieces and fry them at 200 degree Celsius.
2. Place olive oil on the side of the bread slices. Layer the rest of the ingredients on the non-oiled side following the following steps, peach preserves, tomatoes, jack cheese and cooked bacon.
3. Press down the bread to allow it to cook a little bit and peach side down too to allow the bread and the peel to spread evenly.
4. Place the sandwich in an air fryer and cook it for 12 minutes
5. at 393 degrees Fahrenheit.
6. Serve once you are done.

- **Nutrition Info:** Calories 282 Fats 18g, Carbs 18g, Proteins 12g, Sodium: 830 Mg, Potassium: 250mg

63. Easy French Toast Casserole

Servings:6
Cooking Time: 12 Minutes
Ingredients:
- 3 large eggs, beaten
- 1 cup whole milk
- 1 tablespoon pure maple syrup
- 1 teaspoon vanilla extract
- ¼ teaspoon cinnamon
- ¼ teaspoon kosher salt
- 3 cups stale bread cubes

- 1 tablespoon unsalted butter, at room temperature
- In a medium bowl, whisk together the eggs, milk, maple syrup, vanilla extract, cinnamon and salt. Stir in the bread cubes to coat well.

Directions:
1. Grease the bottom of the baking pan with the butter. Spread the bread mixture into the pan in an even layer.
2. Slide the baking pan into Rack Position 2, select Roast, set temperature to 350ºF (180ºC) and set time to 12 minutes.
3. After about 10 minutes, remove the pan and check the casserole. The top should be browned and the middle of the casserole just set. If more time is needed, return the pan to the oven and continue cooking.
4. When cooking is complete, serve warm.

64. Tasty Cheddar Omelet

Servings: 1
Cooking Time: 20 Minutes
Ingredients:
- 2 eggs
- 2 tbsp cheddar cheese, grated
- 1 tsp soy sauce
- ½ onion, sliced
- Salt and black pepper to taste
- 1 tbsp olive oil

Directions:
1. Preheat Breville Smart on Bake function to 350 F. Whisk the eggs with soy sauce, salt, and pepper. Stir in onion. Grease a baking dish with the olive oil and add in the egg mixture. Cook for 10-14 minutes. Top with the grated cheddar cheese and serve.

65. Fried Cheese Grits

Servings:4
Cooking Time: 11 Minutes
Ingredients:
- $^2/_3$ cup instant grits
- 1 teaspoon salt
- 1 teaspoon freshly ground black pepper
- ¾ cup whole or 2% milk
- 3 ounces (85 g) cream cheese, at room temperature
- 1 large egg, beaten

- 1 tablespoon butter, melted
- 1 cup shredded mild Cheddar cheese
- Cooking spray

Directions:
1. Mix the grits, salt, and black pepper in a large bowl. Add the milk, cream cheese, beaten egg, and melted butter and whisk to combine. Fold in the Cheddar cheese and stir well.
2. Spray the baking pan with cooking spray. Spread the grits mixture into the baking pan.
3. Put the air fryer basket on the baking pan and slide into Rack Position 2, select Air Fry, set temperature to 400ºF (205ºC) and set time to 11 minutes.
4. Stir the mixture halfway through the cooking time.
5. When done, a knife inserted in the center should come out clean.
6. Rest for 5 minutes and serve warm.

66. Baja Fish Tacos

Servings: 6 Tacos
Cooking Time: 17 Minutes
Ingredients:
- 1 egg
- 5 ounces (142 g) Mexican beer
- ¾ cup all-purpose flour
- ¾ cup cornstarch
- ¼ teaspoon chili powder
- ½ teaspoon ground cumin
- ½ pound (227 g) cod, cut into large pieces
- 6 corn tortillas
- Cooking spray
- Salsa:
- 1 mango, peeled and diced
- ¼ red bell pepper, diced
- ½ small jalapeño, diced
- ¼ red onion, minced
- Juice of half a lime
- Pinch chopped fresh cilantro
- ¼ teaspoon salt
- ¼ teaspoon ground black pepper

Directions:
1. Spritz the air fryer basket with cooking spray.

2. Whisk the egg with beer in a bowl. Combine the flour, cornstarch, chili powder, and cumin in a separate bowl.
3. Dredge the cod in the egg mixture first, then in the flour mixture to coat well. Shake the excess off.
4. Arrange the cod in the basket and spritz with cooking spray.
5. Put the air fryer basket on the baking pan and slide into Rack Position 2, select Air Fry, set temperature to 380ºF (193ºC) and set time to 17 minutes.
6. Flip the cod halfway through the cooking time.
7. When cooked, the cod should be golden brown and crunchy.
8. Meanwhile, combine the ingredients for the salsa in a small bowl. Stir to mix well.
9. Unfold the tortillas on a clean work surface, then divide the fish on the tortillas and spread the salsa on top. Fold to serve.

67. Breakfast Cheese Sandwiches

Servings:2
Cooking Time: 8 Minutes
Ingredients:
- 1 teaspoon butter, softened
- 4 slices bread
- 4 slices smoked country ham
- 4 slices Cheddar cheese
- 4 thick slices tomato

Directions:
1. Spoon ½ teaspoon of butter onto one side of 2 slices of bread and spread it all over.
2. Assemble the sandwiches: Top each of 2 slices of unbuttered bread with 2 slices of ham, 2 slices of cheese, and 2 slices of tomato. Place the remaining 2 slices of bread on top, butter-side up.
3. Lay the sandwiches in the baking pan, buttered side down.
4. Slide the baking pan into Rack Position 1, select Convection Bake, set temperature to 370ºF (188ºC), and set time to 8 minutes.
5. Flip the sandwiches halfway through the cooking time.
6. When cooking is complete, the sandwiches should be golden brown on both sides and the cheese should be melted. Remove from the oven. Allow to cool for 5 minutes before slicing to serve.

68. Beef And Bell Pepper Fajitas

Servings:4
Cooking Time: 10 Minutes
Ingredients:
- 1 pound (454 g) beef sirloin steak, cut into strips
- 2 shallots, sliced
- 1 orange bell pepper, sliced
- 1 red bell pepper, sliced
- 2 garlic cloves, minced
- 2 tablespoons Cajun seasoning
- 1 tablespoon paprika
- Salt and ground black pepper, to taste
- 4 corn tortillas
- ½ cup shredded Cheddar cheese
- Cooking spray

Directions:
1. Spritz the air fryer basket with cooking spray.
2. Combine all the ingredients, except for the tortillas and cheese, in a large bowl. Toss to coat well.
3. Pour the beef and vegetables in the pan and spritz with cooking spray.
4. Put the air fryer basket on the baking pan and slide into Rack Position 2, select Air Fry, set temperature to 360ºF (182ºC) and set time to 10 minutes.
5. Stir the beef and vegetables halfway through the cooking time.
6. When cooking is complete, the meat will be browned and the vegetables will be soft and lightly wilted.
7. Unfold the tortillas on a clean work surface and spread the cooked beef and vegetables on top. Scatter with cheese and fold to serve.

69. Poppy Seed Muffins

Servings: 12
Cooking Time: 20 Minutes
Ingredients:
- 3 tbsp poppy seeds
- 1 tsp vanilla
- 8 tbsp maple syrup

- 2 tbsp lemon zest
- 6 tbsp lemon juice
- 4/5 cup almond milk
- 1/4 cup butter, melted
- 1/4 tsp baking soda
- 2 tsp baking powder
- 1 1/4 cups flour
- 1 1/4 cups almond flour
- Pinch of salt

Directions:
1. Fit the Breville Smart oven with the rack in position
2. Line 12-cups muffin tin with cupcake liners and set aside.
3. In a large bowl, mix together melted butter, milk, lemon zest, vanilla, lemon juice, poppy seeds, maple syrup, and almond flour.
4. Add flour, baking soda, and baking powder. Stir until well combined.
5. Pour batter into the prepared muffin tin.
6. Set to bake at 350 F for 25 minutes, after 5 minutes, place the muffin tin in the oven.
7. Serve and enjoy.
- **Nutrition Info:** Calories 239 Fat 14.4 g Carbohydrates 23.6 g Sugar 9.1 g Protein 4.7 g Cholesterol 10 mg

70. Cherry Cinnamon Almond Breakfast Scones

Servings:x
Cooking Time:x
Ingredients:
- 2 cups all-purpose flour
- ½ cup chopped almonds
- ¾ cup milk
- ½ tsp cinnamon
- 2 tsp baking powder
- 3 Tbsp brown sugar
- Pinch of salt
- ½ cup cold butter
- 1½ cups dried cherries
- Zest of one lemon
- 2 Tbsp turbinado sugar

Directions:
1. Preheat oven to 375°F.
2. Combine flour, baking powder, brown sugar and salt.

3. Add cold butter, cut into small pieces, and pinch until dough becomes crumbly.
4. Add dried cherries, zest and chopped almonds to combine.
5. Add the milk and mix dough gently. Do not overwork.
6. Grease Breville smart oven and spread dough uniformly.
7. Combine cinnamon and turbinado sugar and sprinkle on top.
8. Bake for about 25 minutes or until scone is cooked through.

71. Delicious French Eggs

Servings: 12
Cooking Time: 10 Minutes
Ingredients:
- 12 eggs
- 1/2 cup heavy cream
- 8 oz parmesan cheese, shredded
- Pepper
- Salt

Directions:
1. Fit the Breville Smart oven with the rack in position
2. Spray 12-cups muffin tin with cooking spray and set aside.
3. Crack each egg into each cup.
4. Divide heavy cream and parmesan cheese evenly into each cup.
5. Season with pepper and salt.
6. Set to bake at 425 F for 15 minutes. After 5 minutes place muffin tin in the preheated oven.
7. Serve and enjoy.
- **Nutrition Info:** Calories 141 Fat 10.3 g Carbohydrates 1.2 g Sugar 0.4 g Protein 11.7 g Cholesterol 184 mg

72. Enchiladas 4 Breakfast

Servings: 8
Cooking Time: 30 Minutes
Ingredients:
- Nonstick cooking spray
- 1 lb. pork breakfast sausage
- 2 cups hash browns, thawed
- 1/3 cup red bell pepper, chopped
- 1/3 cup poblano pepper, chopped

- 6 green onion, sliced thin
- 2 tsp garlic salt divided
- 10 eggs
- 1 tsp black pepper
- 3 cups pepper jack cheese, grated
- 8 8-inch
- 1 cup salsa Verde
- ½ cup half & half
- ½ tsp cumin
- ½ tsp oregano

Directions:
1. Place the rack in position Lightly spray an 8x11-inch baking dish with cooking spray.
2. In a medium saucepan, over medium heat, cook sausage until no longer pink. Use a slotted spoon to transfer to a paper towel lined plate.
3. Add potatoes, red pepper, poblano, 1 teaspoon garlic salt, and onion (saving 3 tablespoons for garnish) to the pan. Cook until vegetables are fork-tender, about 5-7 minutes. Stir in sausage and stir to combine. Remove from heat.
4. In a medium bowl, whisk eggs, remaining garlic salt, and pepper.
5. Heat a medium skillet over medium heat. Once hot, add eggs and scramble until done. Remove from heat.
6. Place tortillas, one at a time, on work surface. Use 2 cups of cheese for filling. Sprinkle some cheese down the middle. Top with sausage mixture and a little more cheese. Roll up and place seam side down in prepared pan. Repeat with remaining ingredients.
7. In a small bowl, whisk together salsa Verde, half & half, cumin, and oregano. Pour over enchiladas and top with remaining cheese.
8. Set to bake on 375°F for 35 minutes. After 5 minutes, place baking pan on rack and bake 30 minutes or until golden brown and bubbly. Serve garnished with reserved onions.
- **Nutrition Info:** Calories 582, Total Fat 36g, Saturated Fat 15g, Total Carbs 31g, Net Carbs 28g, Protein 31g, Sugar 4g, Fiber 3g, Sodium 1015mg, Potassium 677mg, Phosphorus 512mg

73. Quick & Easy Granola

Servings: 4
Cooking Time: 8 Minutes
Ingredients:
- 2 cups oats
- 2 tbsp chia seeds
- 1 tsp vanilla
- 1/2 tsp cinnamon
- 1/4 cup honey
- 1/4 cup almond butter

Directions:
1. Fit the Breville Smart oven with the rack in position
2. In a bowl, mix the almond butter, honey, cinnamon, and vanilla.
3. Add oats and chia seeds and mix well.
4. Transfer oats mixture onto the parchment-lined baking pan.
5. Place the baking pan in Breville Smart oven and set to bake at 350 F for 8 minutes.
6. Serve and enjoy.
- **Nutrition Info:** Calories 248 Fat 4.4 g Carbohydrates 47.3 g Sugar 18 g Protein 6.3 g Cholesterol 6.3 mg

74. Cheesy Baked-egg Toast

Servings: 4
Cooking Time: 10 Minutes
Ingredients:
- 4 slices wheat bread
- 4 eggs
- 1 cup shredded cheese
- 2 tablespoons softened butter

Directions:
1. Start by preheating toaster oven to 350°F.
2. Place bread on a greased baking sheet.
3. Use a teaspoon to push a square into the bread creating a little bed for the egg.
4. Sprinkle salt and pepper over the bread.
5. Break one egg into each square. Spread butter over each edge of the bread.
6. Sprinkle 1/4 cup cheese over buttered area.
7. Bake for 10 minutes or until the eggs are solid and the cheese is golden brown.
- **Nutrition Info:** Calories: 297, Sodium: 410 mg, Dietary Fiber: 1.9 g, Total Fat: 20.4 g, Total Carbs: 12.3 g, Protein: 16.3 g.

75. Broccoli Asparagus Frittata

Servings: 6
Cooking Time: 20 Minutes
Ingredients:
- 6 eggs
- 1/2 cup onion, diced & sautéed
- 1 cup asparagus, chopped & sautéed
- 1 cup broccoli, chopped & sautéed
- 3 bacon slices, cooked & chopped
- 1/3 cup parmesan cheese, grated
- 1/2 cup milk
- 1/2 tsp pepper
- 1 tsp salt

Directions:
1. Fit the Breville Smart oven with the rack in position
2. In a mixing bowl, whisk eggs with milk, cheese, pepper, and salt.
3. Add onion, asparagus, broccoli, and bacon and stir well.
4. Pour egg mixture into the greased baking dish.
5. Set to bake at 350 F for 25 minutes. After 5 minutes place the baking dish in the preheated oven.
6. Serve and enjoy.
- **Nutrition Info:** Calories 154 Fat 9.9 g Carbohydrates 4.6 g Sugar 2.4 g Protein 12.4 g Cholesterol 179 mg

76. Breakfast Oatmeal With Blueberries

Servings:x
Cooking Time:x
Ingredients:
- 1-2 Tbsp butter
- ½ Gala apple, peeled, cored and cut into ½-inch pieces
- Pinch kosher salt
- ⅔ cup whole milk
- 1 egg yolk
- ½ cup fresh blueberries
- 1 Tbsp maple syrup
- ⅔ cup uncooked rolled oats
- ¼ cup blanched slivered almonds
- ¼ tsp baking powder
- ¼ tsp cinnamon
- 2 tsp brown sugar

- ¼ tsp vanilla extract

Directions:
1. Preheat the oven to 375°F.
2. Butter the bottom of Breville smart oven and about 1 inch up the sides.
3. Add the apple and blueberries in a thin layer. Drizzle with the maple syrup.
4. In a medium bowl, mix together the oats, almonds, baking powder, cinnamon, and salt.
5. In a small bowl, whisk together the milk, egg yolk, sugar, and vanilla and pour over the oat mixture. Stir just until combined and spoon over the fruit.
6. Bake, uncovered, for 30 to 35 minutes, or until the top is golden brown and the fruit is bubbling. Let cool for 10 to 15 minutes before serving.

77. Meat Lover Omelet With Mozzarella

Servings:2
Cooking Time: 20 Minutes
Ingredients:
- 1 beef sausage, chopped
- 4 slices prosciutto, chopped
- 3 oz salami, chopped
- 1 cup grated mozzarella cheese
- 4 eggs
- 1 tbsp chopped onion
- 1 tbsp ketchup

Directions:
1. Preheat Breville on Bake function to 350 F. Whisk the eggs with ketchup in a bowl. Stir in the onion. Brown the sausage in a greased pan over medium heat for 2 minutes.
2. Combine the egg mixture, mozzarella cheese, salami, and prosciutto. Pour the egg mixture over the sausage and give it a stir. Press Start and cook in the Breville for 15 minutes.

78. Turkey Sliders With Chive Mayo

Servings:6
Cooking Time: 15 Minutes
Ingredients:
- 12 burger buns
- Cooking spray

- Turkey Sliders:
- ¾ pound (340 g) turkey, minced
- 1 tablespoon oyster sauce
- ¼ cup pickled jalapeno, chopped
- 2 tablespoons chopped scallions
- 1 tablespoon chopped fresh cilantro
- 1 to 2 cloves garlic, minced
- Sea salt and ground black pepper, to taste
- Chive Mayo:
- 1 tablespoon chives
- 1 cup mayonnaise
- Zest of 1 lime
- 1 teaspoon salt

Directions:

1. Spritz the air fryer basket with cooking spray.
2. Combine the ingredients for the turkey sliders in a large bowl. Stir to mix well. Shape the mixture into 6 balls, then bash the balls into patties.
3. Arrange the patties in the pan and spritz with cooking spray.
4. Put the air fryer basket on the baking pan and slide into Rack Position 2, select Air Fry, set temperature to 365ºF (185ºC) and set time to 15 minutes.
5. Flip the patties halfway through the cooking time.
6. Meanwhile, combine the ingredients for the chive mayo in a small bowl. Stir to mix well.
7. When cooked, the patties will be well browned.
8. Smear the patties with chive mayo, then assemble the patties between two buns to make the sliders. Serve immediately.

LUNCH RECIPES

79. Sweet Potato Rosti

Servings: 2
Cooking Time: 15 Minutes
Ingredients:
- ½ lb. sweet potatoes, peeled, grated and squeezed
- 1 tablespoon fresh parsley, chopped finely
- Salt and ground black pepper, as required
- 2 tablespoons sour cream

Directions:
1. In a large bowl, mix together the grated sweet potato, parsley, salt, and black pepper.
2. Press "Power Button" of Air Fry Oven and turn the dial to select the "Air Fry" mode.
3. Press the Time button and again turn the dial to set the cooking time to 15 minutes.
4. Now push the Temp button and rotate the dial to set the temperature at 355 degrees F.
5. Press "Start/Pause" button to start.
6. When the unit beeps to show that it is preheated, open the lid and lightly, grease the sheet pan.
7. Arrange the sweet potato mixture into the "Sheet Pan" and shape it into an even circle.
8. Insert the "Sheet Pan" in the oven.
9. Cut the potato rosti into wedges.
10. Top with the sour cream and serve immediately.
- **Nutrition Info:** Calories: 160 Cal Total Fat: 2.7 g Saturated Fat: 1.6 g Cholesterol: 5 mg Sodium: 95 mg Total Carbs: 32.3 g Fiber: 4.7 g Sugar: 0.6 g Protein: 2.2 g

80. Turkey Meatballs With Manchego Cheese

Servings: 4
Cooking Time: 10 Minutes
Ingredients:
- 1 pound ground turkey
- 1/2 pound ground pork
- 1 egg, well beaten
- 1 teaspoon dried basil
- 1 teaspoon dried rosemary
- 1/4 cup Manchego cheese, grated
- 2 tablespoons yellow onions, finely chopped
- 1 teaspoon fresh garlic, finely chopped
- Sea salt and ground black pepper, to taste

Directions:
1. In a mixing bowl, combine all the ingredients until everything is well incorporated.
2. Shape the mixture into 1-inch balls.
3. Cook the meatballs in the preheated Air Fryer at 380 degrees for 7 minutes. Shake halfway through the cooking time. Work in batches.
4. Serve with your favorite pasta.
- **Nutrition Info:** 386 Calories; 24g Fat; 9g Carbs; 41g Protein; 3g Sugars; 2g Fiber

81. Chicken With Veggies And Rice

Servings: 3
Cooking Time: 20 Minutes
Ingredients:
- 3 cups cold boiled white rice
- 1 cup cooked chicken, diced
- ½ cup frozen carrots
- ½ cup frozen peas
- ½ cup onion, chopped
- 6 tablespoons soy sauce
- 1 tablespoon vegetable oil

Directions:
1. Preheat the Air fryer to 360 degree F and grease a 7" nonstick pan.
2. Mix the rice, soy sauce, and vegetable oil in a bowl.
3. Stir in the remaining ingredients and mix until well combined.
4. Transfer the rice mixture into the pan and place in the Air fryer.
5. Cook for about 20 minutes and dish out to serve immediately.
- **Nutrition Info:** Calories: 405, Fat: 6.4g, Carbohydrates: 63g, Sugar: 3.5g, Protein: 21.7g, Sodium: 1500mg

82. Beef Steaks With Beans

Servings: 4
Cooking Time: 10 Minutes
Ingredients:
- 4 beef steaks, trim the fat and cut into strips
- 1 cup green onions, chopped

- 2 cloves garlic, minced
- 1 red bell pepper, seeded and thinly sliced
- 1 can tomatoes, crushed
- 1 can cannellini beans
- 3/4 cup beef broth
- 1/4 teaspoon dried basil
- 1/2 teaspoon cayenne pepper
- 1/2 teaspoon sea salt
- 1/4 teaspoon ground black pepper, or to taste

Directions:

1. Preparing the ingredients. Add the steaks, green onions and garlic to the instant crisp air fryer basket.
2. Air frying. Close air fryer lid. Cook at 390 degrees f for 10 minutes, working in batches.
3. Stir in the remaining ingredients and cook for an additional 5 minutes.
- **Nutrition Info:** Calories 284 Total fat 7.9 g Saturated fat 1.4 g Cholesterol 36 mg Sodium 704 mg Total carbs 46 g Fiber 3.6 g Sugar 5.5 g Protein 17.9 g

83. Herbed Radish Sauté(3)

Servings: 4
Cooking Time: 12 Minutes
Ingredients:

- 2 bunches red radishes; halved
- 2 tbsp. parsley; chopped.
- 2 tbsp. balsamic vinegar
- 1 tbsp. olive oil
- Salt and black pepper to taste.

Directions:

1. Take a bowl and mix the radishes with the remaining ingredients except the parsley, toss and put them in your air fryer's basket.
2. Cook at 400°F for 15 minutes, divide between plates, sprinkle the parsley on top and serve as a side dish
- **Nutrition Info:** Calories: 180; Fat: 4g; Fiber: 2g; Carbs: 3g; Protein: 5g

84. Herb-roasted Turkey Breast

Servings: 8
Cooking Time: 60 Minutes
Ingredients:

- 3 lb turkey breast

- Rub Ingredients:
- 2 tbsp olive oil
- 2 tbsp lemon juice
- 1 tbsp minced Garlic
- 2 tsp ground mustard
- 2 tsp kosher salt
- 1 tsp pepper
- 1 tsp dried rosemary
- 1 tsp dried thyme
- 1 tsp ground sage

Directions:

1. Take a small bowl and thoroughly combine the Rub Ingredients: in it. Rub this on the outside of the turkey breast and under any loose skin.
2. Place the coated turkey breast keeping skin side up on a cooking tray.
3. Place the drip pan at the bottom of the cooking chamber of the Instant Pot Duo Crisp Air Fryer. Select Air Fry option, post this, adjust the temperature to 360°F and the time to one hour, then touch start.
4. When preheated, add the food to the cooking tray in the lowest position. Close the lid for cooking.
5. When the Air Fry program is complete, check to make sure that the thickest portion of the meat reads at least 160°F, remove the turkey and let it rest for 10 minutes before slicing and serving.
- **Nutrition Info:** Calories 214, Total Fat 10g, Total Carbs 2g, Protein 29g

85. Baked Shrimp Scampi

Servings: 4
Cooking Time: 10 Minutes
Ingredients:

- 1 lb large shrimp
- 8 tbsp butter
- 1 tbsp minced garlic (use 2 for extra garlic flavor)
- 1/4 cup white wine or cooking sherry
- 1/2 tsp salt
- 1/4 tsp cayenne pepper
- 1/4 tsp paprika
- 1/2 tsp onion powder
- 3/4 cup bread crumbs

Directions:

1. Take a bowl and mix the bread crumbs with dry seasonings.
2. On the stovetop (or in the Instant Pot on saute), melt the butter with the garlic and the white wine.
3. Remove from heat and add the shrimp and the bread crumb mix.
4. Transfer the mix to a casserole dish.
5. Choose the Bake operation and add food to the Instant Pot Duo Crisp Air Fryer. Close the lid and Bake at 350°F for 10 minutes or until they are browned.
6. Serve and enjoy.
- **Nutrition Info:** Calories 422, Total Fat 26g, Total Carbs 18g, Protein 29 g

86. Mushroom Meatloaf

Servings: 4
Cooking Time: 25 Minutes
Ingredients:
- 14-ounce lean ground beef
- 1 chorizo sausage, chopped finely
- 1 small onion, chopped
- 1 garlic clove, minced
- 2 tablespoons fresh cilantro, chopped
- 3 tablespoons breadcrumbs
- 1 egg
- Salt and freshly ground black pepper, to taste
- 2 tablespoons fresh mushrooms, sliced thinly
- 3 tablespoons olive oil

Directions:
1. Preparing the ingredients. Preheat the instant crisp air fryer to 390 degrees f.
2. In a large bowl, add all ingredients except mushrooms and mix till well combined.
3. In a baking pan, place the beef mixture.
4. With the back of spatula, smooth the surface.
5. Top with mushroom slices and gently, press into the meatloaf.
6. Drizzle with oil evenly.
7. Air frying. Arrange the pan in the instant crisp air fryer basket, close air fryer lid and cook for about 25 minutes.
8. Cut the meatloaf in desires size wedges and serve.

- **Nutrition Info:** Calories 284 Total fat 7.9 g Saturated fat 1.4 g Cholesterol 36 mg Sodium 704 mg Total carbs 46 g Fiber 3.6 g Sugar 5.5 g Protein 17.9 g

87. Simple Turkey Breast

Servings: 10
Cooking Time: 40 Minutes
Ingredients:
- 1: 8-poundsbone-in turkey breast
- Salt and black pepper, as required
- 2 tablespoons olive oil

Directions:
1. Preheat the Air fryer to 360 degree F and grease an Air fryer basket.
2. Season the turkey breast with salt and black pepper and drizzle with oil.
3. Arrange the turkey breast into the Air Fryer basket, skin side down and cook for about 20 minutes.
4. Flip the side and cook for another 20 minutes.
5. Dish out in a platter and cut into desired size slices to serve.

- **Nutrition Info:** Calories: 719, Fat: 35.9g, Carbohydrates: 0g, Sugar: 0g, Protein: 97.2g, Sodium: 386mg

88. Simple Lamb Bbq With Herbed Salt

Servings: 8
Cooking Time: 1 Hour 20 Minutes
Ingredients:
- 2 ½ tablespoons herb salt
- 2 tablespoons olive oil
- 4 pounds boneless leg of lamb, cut into 2-inch chunks

Directions:
1. Preheat the air fryer to 390 ºF.
2. Place the grill pan accessory in the air fryer.
3. Season the meat with the herb salt and brush with olive oil.
4. Grill the meat for 20 minutes per batch.
5. Make sure to flip the meat every 10 minutes for even cooking.

- **Nutrition Info:** Calories: 347 kcal Total Fat: 17.8 g Saturated Fat: 0 g Cholesterol: 0 mg Sodium: 0 mg Total Carbs: 0 g Fiber: 0 g Sugar: 0 g Protein: 46.6 g

89. Parmesan-crusted Pork Loin

Servings: 4
Cooking Time: 20 Minutes
Ingredients:
- 1 pound pork loin
- 1 teaspoon salt
- 1/2 tablespoon garlic powder
- 1/2 tablespoon onion powder
- 2 tablespoons parmesan cheese
- 1 tablespoon olive oil

Directions:
1. Start by preheating toaster oven to 475°F.
2. Place pan in the oven and let it heat while the oven preheats.
3. Mix all ingredients in a shallow dish and roll the pork loin until it is fully coated.
4. Remove pan and sear the pork in the pan on each side.
5. Once seared, bake pork in the pan for 20 minutes.
- **Nutrition Info:** Calories: 334, Sodium: 718 mg, Dietary Fiber: 0 g, Total Fat: 20.8 g, Total Carbs: 1.7 g, Protein: 33.5 g.

90. Glazed Lamb Chops

Servings: 4
Cooking Time: 15 Minutes
Ingredients:
- 1 tablespoon Dijon mustard
- ½ tablespoon fresh lime juice
- 1 teaspoon honey
- ½ teaspoon olive oil
- Salt and ground black pepper, as required
- 4 (4-ounce) lamb loin chops

Directions:
1. In a black pepper large bowl, mix together the mustard, lemon juice, oil, honey, salt, and black pepper.
2. Add the chops and coat with the mixture generously.
3. Place the chops onto the greased "Sheet Pan".
4. Press "Power Button" of Ninja Foodi Digital Air Fry Oven and turn the dial to select the "Air Bake" mode.
5. Press the Time button and again turn the dial to set the cooking time to 15 minutes.

6. Now push the Temp button and rotate the dial to set the temperature at 390 degrees F.
7. Press "Start/Pause" button to start.
8. When the unit beeps to show that it is preheated, open the lid.
9. Insert the "Sheet Pan" in oven.
10. Flip the chops once halfway through.
11. Serve hot.
- **Nutrition Info:** Calories: 224 kcal Total Fat: 9.1 g Saturated Fat: 3.1 g Cholesterol: 102 mg Sodium: 169 mg Total Carbs: 1.7 g Fiber: 0.1 g Sugar: 1.5 g Protein: 32 g

91. Garlic Chicken Potatoes

Servings: 4
Cooking Time: 30 Minutes
Ingredients:
- 2 lbs. red potatoes, quartered
- 3 tablespoons olive oil
- 1/2 teaspoon cumin seeds
- Salt and black pepper, to taste
- 4 garlic cloves, chopped
- 2 tablespoons brown sugar
- 1 lemon (1/2 juiced and 1/2 cut into wedges)
- Pinch of red pepper flakes
- 4 skinless, boneless chicken breasts
- 2 tablespoons cilantro, chopped

Directions:
1. Place the chicken, lemon, garlic, and potatoes in a baking pan.
2. Toss the spices, herbs, oil, and sugar in a bowl.
3. Add this mixture to the chicken and veggies then toss well to coat.
4. Press "Power Button" of Air Fry Oven and turn the dial to select the "Bake" mode.
5. Press the Time button and again turn the dial to set the cooking time to 30 minutes.
6. Now push the Temp button and rotate the dial to set the temperature at 400 degrees F.
7. Once preheated, place the baking pan inside and close its lid.
8. Serve warm.
- **Nutrition Info:** Calories 545 Total Fat 36.4 g Saturated Fat 10.1 g Cholesterol 200 mg Sodium 272 mg Total Carbs 40.7 g Fiber 0.2 g Sugar 0.1 g Protein 42.5 g

92. Bok Choy And Butter Sauce(1)

Servings: 4
Cooking Time: 12 Minutes
Ingredients:
- 2 bok choy heads; trimmed and cut into strips
- 1 tbsp. butter; melted
- 2 tbsp. chicken stock
- 1 tsp. lemon juice
- 1 tbsp. olive oil
- A pinch of salt and black pepper

Directions:
1. In a pan that fits your air fryer, mix all the ingredients, toss, introduce the pan in the air fryer and cook at 380°F for 15 minutes.
2. Divide between plates and serve as a side dish
- **Nutrition Info:** Calories: 141; Fat: 3g; Fiber: 2g; Carbs: 4g; Protein: 3g

93. Deviled Chicken

Servings: 8
Cooking Time: 40 Minutes
Ingredients:
- 2 tablespoons butter
- 2 cloves garlic, chopped
- 1 cup Dijon mustard
- 1/2 teaspoon cayenne pepper
- 1 1/2 cups panko breadcrumbs
- 3/4 cup Parmesan, freshly grated
- 1/4 cup chives, chopped
- 2 teaspoons paprika
- 8 small bone-in chicken thighs, skin removed

Directions:
1. Toss the chicken thighs with crumbs, cheese, chives, butter, and spices in a bowl and mix well to coat.
2. Transfer the chicken along with its spice mix to a baking pan.
3. Press "Power Button" of Air Fry Oven and turn the dial to select the "Air Fry" mode.
4. Press the Time button and again turn the dial to set the cooking time to 40 minutes.
5. Now push the Temp button and rotate the dial to set the temperature at 350 degrees F.

6. Once preheated, place the baking pan inside and close its lid.
7. Serve warm.
- **Nutrition Info:** Calories 380 Total Fat 20 g Saturated Fat 5 g Cholesterol 151 mg Sodium 686 mg Total Carbs 33 g Fiber 1 g Sugar 1.2 g Protein 21 g

94. Juicy Turkey Burgers

Servings: 8
Cooking Time: 25 Minutes
Ingredients:
- 1 lb ground turkey 85% lean / 15% fat
- ¼ cup unsweetened apple sauce
- ½ onion grated
- 1 Tbsp ranch seasoning
- 2 tsp Worcestershire Sauce
- 1 tsp minced garlic
- ¼ cup plain breadcrumbs
- Salt and pepper to taste

Directions:
1. Combine the onion, ground turkey, unsweetened apple sauce, minced garlic, breadcrumbs, ranch seasoning, Worchestire sauce, and salt and pepper. Mix them with your hands until well combined. Form 4 equally sized hamburger patties with them.
2. Place these burgers in the refrigerator for about 30 minutes to have them firm up a bit.
3. While preparing for cooking, select the Air Fry option. Set the temperature of 360°F and the cook time as required. Press start to begin preheating.
4. Once the preheating temperature is reached, place the burgers on the tray in the Air fryer basket, making sure they don't overlap or touch. Cook on for 15 minutes
5. flipping halfway through.
- **Nutrition Info:** Calories 183, Total Fat 3g, Total Carbs 11g, Protein 28g

95. Turkey And Almonds

Servings: 2
Cooking Time: 10 Minutes
Ingredients:
- 1 big turkey breast, skinless; boneless and halved
- 2 shallots; chopped

- 1/3 cup almonds; chopped
- 1 tbsp. sweet paprika
- 2 tbsp. olive oil
- Salt and black pepper to taste.

Directions:

1. In a pan that fits the air fryer, combine the turkey with all the other ingredients, toss.
2. Put the pan in the machine and cook at 370°F for 25 minutes
3. Divide everything between plates and serve.
- **Nutrition Info:** Calories: 274; Fat: 12g; Fiber: 3g; Carbs: 5g; Protein: 14g

96. Lamb Gyro

Servings: 4
Cooking Time: 25 Minutes
Ingredients:

- 1 pound ground lamb
- ¼ red onion, minced
- ¼ cup mint, minced
- ¼ cup parsley, minced
- 2 cloves garlic, minced
- ½ teaspoon salt
- ⅛ teaspoon rosemary
- ½ teaspoon black pepper
- 4 slices pita bread
- ¾ cup hummus
- 1 cup romaine lettuce, shredded
- ½ onion sliced
- 1 Roma tomato, diced
- ½ cucumber, skinned and thinly sliced
- 12 mint leaves, minced
- Tzatziki sauce, to taste

Directions:

1. Mix ground lamb, red onion, mint, parsley, garlic, salt, rosemary, and black pepper until fully incorporated.
2. Select the Broil function on the COSORI Air Fryer Toaster Oven, set time to 25 minutes and temperature to 450°F, then press Start/Cancel to preheat.
3. Line the food tray with parchment paper and place ground lamb on top, shaping it into a patty 1-inch-thick and 6 inches in diameter.
4. Insert the food tray at top position in the preheated air fryer toaster oven, then press Start/Cancel.
5. Remove when done and cut into thin slices.
6. Assemble each gyro starting with pita bread, then hummus, lamb meat, lettuce, onion, tomato, cucumber, and mint leaves, then drizzle with tzatziki.
7. Serve immediately.
- **Nutrition Info:** Calories: 409 kcal Total Fat: 14.6 g Saturated Fat: 0 g Cholesterol: 0 mg Sodium: 0 mg Total Carbs: 29.9 g Fiber: 0 g Sugar: 0 g Protein: 39.4 g

97. Onion Omelet

Servings: 2
Cooking Time: 15 Minutes
Ingredients:

- 4 eggs
- ¼ teaspoon low-sodium soy sauce
- Ground black pepper, as required
- 1 teaspoon butter
- 1 medium yellow onion, sliced
- ¼ cup Cheddar cheese, grated

Directions:

1. In a skillet, melt the butter over medium heat and cook the onion and cook for about 8-10 minutes.
2. Remove from the heat and set aside to cool slightly.
3. Meanwhile, in a bowl, add the eggs, soy sauce and black pepper and beat well.
4. Add the cooked onion and gently, stir to combine.
5. Place the zucchini mixture into a small baking pan.
6. Press "Power Button" of Air Fry Oven and turn the dial to select the "Air Fry" mode.
7. Press the Time button and again turn the dial to set the cooking time to 5 minutes.
8. Now push the Temp button and rotate the dial to set the temperature at 355 degrees F.
9. Press "Start/Pause" button to start.
10. When the unit beeps to show that it is preheated, open the lid.
11. Arrange pan over the "Wire Rack" and insert in the oven.
12. Cut the omelet into 2 portions and serve hot.
- **Nutrition Info:** Calories: 222 Cal Total Fat: 15.4 g Saturated Fat: 6.9 g Cholesterol: 347

mg Sodium: 264 mg Total Carbs: 6.1 g Fiber: 1.2 g Sugar: 3.1 g Protein: 15.3 g

98. Ricotta Toasts With Salmon

Servings: 2
Cooking Time: 4 Minutes
Ingredients:
- 4 bread slices
- 1 garlic clove, minced
- 8 oz. ricotta cheese
- 1 teaspoon lemon zest
- Freshly ground black pepper, to taste
- 4 oz. smoked salmon

Directions:
1. In a food processor, add the garlic, ricotta, lemon zest and black pepper and pulse until smooth.
2. Spread ricotta mixture over each bread slices evenly.
3. Press "Power Button" of Air Fry Oven and turn the dial to select the "Air Fry" mode.
4. Press the Time button and again turn the dial to set the cooking time to 4 minutes.
5. Now push the Temp button and rotate the dial to set the temperature at 355 degrees F.
6. Press "Start/Pause" button to start.
7. When the unit beeps to show that it is preheated, open the lid and lightly, grease the sheet pan.
8. Arrange the bread slices into "Air Fry Basket" and insert in the oven.
9. Top with salmon and serve.
- **Nutrition Info:** Calories: 274 Cal Total Fat: 12 g Saturated Fat: 6.3 g Cholesterol: 48 mg Sodium: 1300 mg Total Carbs: 15.7 g Fiber: 0.5 g Sugar: 1.2 g Protein: 24.8 g

99. Roasted Grape And Goat Cheese Crostinis

Servings: 10
Cooking Time: 5 Minutes
Ingredients:
- 1 pound seedless red grapes
- 1 teaspoon chopped rosemary
- 4 tablespoons olive oil
- 1 rustic French baguette
- 1 cup sliced shallots
- 2 tablespoons unsalted butter
- 8 ounces goat cheese
- 1 tablespoon honey

Directions:
1. Start by preheating toaster oven to 400°F.
2. Toss grapes, rosemary, and 1 tablespoon of olive oil in a large bowl.
3. Transfer to a roasting pan and roast for 20 minutes.
4. Remove the pan from the oven and set aside to cool.
5. Slice the baguette into 1/2-inch-thick pieces.
6. Brush each slice with olive oil and place on baking sheet.
7. Bake for 8 minutes, then remove from oven and set aside.
8. In a medium skillet add butter and one tablespoon of olive oil.
9. Add shallots and sauté for about 10 minutes.
10. Mix goat cheese and honey in a medium bowl, then add contents of shallot pan and mix thoroughly.
11. Spread shallot mixture onto baguette, top with grapes, and serve.
- **Nutrition Info:** Calories: 238, Sodium: 139 mg, Dietary Fiber: 0.6 g, Total Fat: 16.3 g, Total Carbs: 16.4 g, Protein: 8.4 g.

100. Chicken Parmesan

Servings: 4
Cooking Time: 10 Minutes
Ingredients:
- 2 (6-oz.boneless, skinless chicken breasts
- 1 oz. pork rinds, crushed
- ½ cup grated Parmesan cheese, divided.
- 1 cup low-carb, no-sugar-added pasta sauce.
- 1 cup shredded mozzarella cheese, divided.
- 4 tbsp. full-fat mayonnaise, divided.
- ½ tsp. garlic powder.
- ¼ tsp. dried oregano.
- ½ tsp. dried parsley.

Directions:
1. Slice each chicken breast in half lengthwise and lb. out to 3/4-inch thickness. Sprinkle with garlic powder, oregano and parsley
2. Spread 1 tbsp. mayonnaise on top of each piece of chicken, then sprinkle ¼ cup mozzarella on each piece.

3. In a small bowl, mix the crushed pork rinds and Parmesan. Sprinkle the mixture on top of mozzarella
4. Pour sauce into 6-inch round baking pan and place chicken on top. Place pan into the air fryer basket. Adjust the temperature to 320 Degrees F and set the timer for 25 minutes
5. Cheese will be browned and internal temperature of the chicken will be at least 165 Degrees F when fully cooked. Serve warm.
- **Nutrition Info:** Calories: 393; Protein: 32g; Fiber: 1g; Fat: 28g; Carbs: 8g

101.Buttermilk Brined Turkey Breast

Servings: 8
Cooking Time: 20 Minutes
Ingredients:
- ¾ cup brine from a can of olives
- 3½ pounds boneless, skinless turkey breast
- 2 fresh thyme sprigs
- 1 fresh rosemary sprig
- ½ cup buttermilk

Directions:
1. Preheat the Air fryer to 350 degree F and grease an Air fryer basket.
2. Mix olive brine and buttermilk in a bowl until well combined.
3. Place the turkey breast, buttermilk mixture and herb sprigs in a resealable plastic bag.
4. Seal the bag and refrigerate for about 12 hours.
5. Remove the turkey breast from bag and arrange the turkey breast into the Air fryer basket.
6. Cook for about 20 minutes, flipping once in between.
7. Dish out the turkey breast onto a cutting board and cut into desired size slices to serve.
- **Nutrition Info:** Calories: 215, Fat: 3.5g, Carbohydrates: 9.4g, Sugar: 7.7g, Protein: 34.4g, Sodium: 2000mg

102.Chicken Breasts With Chimichurri

Servings: 1
Cooking Time: 35 Minutes

Ingredients:
- 1 chicken breast, bone-in, skin-on
- Chimichurri
- ½ bunch fresh cilantro
- 1/4 bunch fresh parsley
- ½ shallot, peeled, cut in quarters
- ½ tablespoon paprika ground
- ½ tablespoon chili powder
- ½ tablespoon fennel ground
- ½ teaspoon black pepper, ground
- ½ teaspoon onion powder
- 1 teaspoon salt
- ½ teaspoon garlic powder
- ½ teaspoon cumin ground
- ½ tablespoon canola oil
- Chimichurri
- 2 tablespoons olive oil
- 4 garlic cloves, peeled
- Zest and juice of 1 lemon
- 1 teaspoon kosher salt

Directions:
1. Preheat the Air fryer to 300 degree F and grease an Air fryer basket.
2. Combine all the spices in a suitable bowl and season the chicken with it.
3. Sprinkle with canola oil and arrange the chicken in the Air fryer basket.
4. Cook for about 35 minutes and dish out in a platter.
5. Put all the ingredients in the blender and blend until smooth.
6. Serve the chicken with chimichurri sauce.
- **Nutrition Info:** Calories: 140, Fats: 7.9g, Carbohydrates: 1.8g, Sugar: 7.1g, Proteins: 7.2g, Sodium: 581mg

103.Persimmon Toast With Sour Cream & Cinnamon

Servings: 1
Cooking Time: 5 Minutes
Ingredients:
- 1 slice of wheat bread
- 1/2 persimmon
- Sour cream to taste
- Sugar to taste
- Cinnamon to taste
Directions:

1. Spread a thin layer of sour cream across the bread.
2. Slice the persimmon into 1/4 inch pieces and lay them across the bread.
3. Sprinkle cinnamon and sugar over persimmon.
4. Toast in toaster oven until bread and persimmon begin to brown.
- **Nutrition Info:** Calories: 89, Sodium: 133 mg, Dietary Fiber: 2.0 g, Total Fat: 1.1 g, Total Carbs: 16.5 g, Protein: 3.8 g.

104.Duck Rolls

Servings: 3
Cooking Time: 40 Minutes
Ingredients:
- 1 pound duck breast fillet, each cut into 2 pieces
- 3 tablespoons fresh parsley, finely chopped
- 1 small red onion, finely chopped
- 1 garlic clove, crushed
- 1½ teaspoons ground cumin
- 1 teaspoon ground cinnamon
- ½ teaspoon red chili powder
- Salt, to taste
- 2 tablespoons olive oil

Directions:
1. Preheat the Air fryer to 355 degree F and grease an Air fryer basket.
2. Mix the garlic, parsley, onion, spices, and 1 tablespoon of olive oil in a bowl.
3. Make a slit in each duck piece horizontally and coat with onion mixture.
4. Roll each duck piece tightly and transfer into the Air fryer basket.
5. Cook for about 40 minutes and cut into desired size slices to serve.
- **Nutrition Info:** Calories: 239, Fats: 8.2g, Carbohydrates: 3.2g, Sugar: 0.9g, Proteins: 37.5g, Sodium: 46mg

105.Chili Chicken Sliders

Servings: 4
Cooking Time: 10 Minutes
Ingredients:
- 1/3 teaspoon paprika
- 1/3 cup scallions, peeled and chopped
- 3 cloves garlic, peeled and minced

- 1 teaspoon ground black pepper, or to taste
- 1/2 teaspoon fresh basil, minced
- 1 ½ cups chicken,minced
- 1 ½ tablespoons coconut aminos
- 1/2 teaspoon grated fresh ginger
- 1/2 tablespoon chili sauce
- 1 teaspoon salt

Directions:
1. Thoroughly combine all ingredients in a mixing dish. Then, form into 4 patties.
2. Cook in the preheated Air Fryer for 18 minutes at 355 degrees F.
3. Garnish with toppings of choice.
- **Nutrition Info:** 366 Calories; 6g Fat; 4g Carbs; 66g Protein; 3g Sugars; 9g Fiber

106.Zucchini And Cauliflower Stew

Servings: 4
Cooking Time: 12 Minutes
Ingredients:
- 1 cauliflower head, florets separated
- 1 ½ cups zucchinis; sliced
- 1 handful parsley leaves; chopped.
- ½ cup tomato puree
- 2 green onions; chopped.
- 1 tbsp. balsamic vinegar
- 1 tbsp. olive oil
- Salt and black pepper to taste.

Directions:
1. In a pan that fits your air fryer, mix the zucchinis with the rest of the ingredients except the parsley, toss, introduce the pan in the air fryer and cook at 380°F for 20 minutes
2. Divide into bowls and serve for lunch with parsley sprinkled on top.
- **Nutrition Info:** Calories: 193; Fat: 5g; Fiber: 2g; Carbs: 4g; Protein: 7g

107.Chicken Caprese Sandwich

Servings: 2
Cooking Time: 3 Minutes
Ingredients:
- 2 leftover chicken breasts, or pre-cooked breaded chicken
- 1 large ripe tomato
- 4 ounces mozzarella cheese slices
- 4 slices of whole grain bread

- 1/4 cup olive oil
- 1/3 cup fresh basil leaves
- Salt and pepper to taste

Directions:
1. Start by slicing tomatoes into thin slices.
2. Layer tomatoes then cheese over two slices of bread and place on a greased baking sheet.
3. Toast in the toaster oven for about 2 minutes or until the cheese is melted.
4. Heat chicken while the cheese melts.
5. Remove from oven, sprinkle with basil, and add chicken.
6. Drizzle with oil and add salt and pepper.
7. Top with other slice of bread and serve.
- **Nutrition Info:** Calories: 808, Sodium: 847 mg, Dietary Fiber: 5.2 g, Total Fat: 43.6 g, Total Carbs: 30.7 g, Protein: 78.4 g.

108.Tomato Frittata

Servings: 2
Cooking Time: 30 Minutes
Ingredients:
- 4 eggs
- ¼ cup onion, chopped
- ½ cup tomatoes, chopped
- ½ cup milk
- 1 cup Gouda cheese, shredded
- Salt, as required

Directions:
1. In a small baking pan, add all the ingredients and mix well.
2. Press "Power Button" of Air Fry Oven and turn the dial to select the "Air Fry" mode.
3. Press the Time button and again turn the dial to set the cooking time to 30 minutes.
4. Now push the Temp button and rotate the dial to set the temperature at 340 degrees F.
5. Press "Start/Pause" button to start.
6. When the unit beeps to show that it is preheated, open the lid.
7. Arrange the baking pan over the "Wire Rack" and insert in the oven.
8. Cut into 2 wedges and serve.
- **Nutrition Info:** Calories: 247 Cal Total Fat: 16.1 g Saturated Fat: 7.5 g Cholesterol: 332 mg Sodium: 417 mg Total Carbs: 7.30 g Fiber: 0.9 g Sugar: 5.2 g Protein: 18.6 g

109.Portobello Pesto Burgers

Servings: 4

Cooking Time: 26 Minutes
Ingredients:
- 4 portobello mushrooms
- 1/4 cup sundried tomato pesto
- 4 whole-grain hamburger buns
- 1 large ripe tomato
- 1 log fresh goat cheese
- 8 large fresh basil leaves

Directions:
1. Start by preheating toaster oven to 425°F.
2. Place mushrooms on a pan, round sides facing up.
3. Bake for 14 minutes.
4. Pull out tray, flip the mushrooms and spread 1 tablespoon of pesto on each piece.
5. Return to oven and bake for another 10 minutes.
6. Remove the mushrooms and toast the buns for 2 minutes.
7. Remove the buns and build the burger by placing tomatoes, mushroom, 2 slices of cheese, and a sprinkle of basil, then topping with the top bun.
- **Nutrition Info:** Calories: 297, Sodium: 346 mg, Dietary Fiber: 1.8 g, Total Fat: 18.1 g, Total Carbs: 19.7 g, Protein: 14.4 g.

110.Perfect Size French Fries

Servings: 1
Cooking Time: 30 Minutes
Ingredients:
- 1 medium potato
- 1 tablespoon olive oil
- Salt and pepper to taste

Directions:
1. Start by preheating your oven to 425°F.
2. Clean the potato and cut it into fries or wedges.
3. Place fries in a bowl of cold water to rinse.
4. Lay the fries on a thick sheet of paper towels and pat dry.
5. Toss in a bowl with oil, salt, and pepper.
6. Bake for 30 minutes.
- **Nutrition Info:** Calories: 284, Sodium: 13 mg, Dietary Fiber: 4.7 g, Total Fat: 14.2 g, Total Carbs: 37.3 g, Protein: 4.3 g.

111.Herbed Duck Legs

Servings: 2
Cooking Time: 30 Minutes
Ingredients:

- ½ tablespoon fresh thyme, chopped
- ½ tablespoon fresh parsley, chopped
- 2 duck legs
- 1 garlic clove, minced
- 1 teaspoon five spice powder
- Salt and black pepper, as required

Directions:

1. Preheat the Air fryer to 340 degree F and grease an Air fryer basket.
2. Mix the garlic, herbs, five spice powder, salt, and black pepper in a bowl.
3. Rub the duck legs with garlic mixture generously and arrange into the Air fryer basket.
4. Cook for about 25 minutes and set the Air fryer to 390 degree F.
5. Cook for 5 more minutes and dish out to serve hot.

- **Nutrition Info:** Calories: 138, Fat: 4.5g, Carbohydrates: 1g, Sugar: 0g, Protein: 25g, Sodium: 82mg

112.Roasted Garlic(2)

Servings: 12 Cloves
Cooking Time: 12 Minutes
Ingredients:

- 1 medium head garlic
- 2 tsp. avocado oil

Directions:

1. Remove any hanging excess peel from the garlic but leave the cloves covered. Cut off ¼ of the head of garlic, exposing the tips of the cloves
2. Drizzle with avocado oil. Place the garlic head into a small sheet of aluminum foil, completely enclosing it. Place it into the air fryer basket. Adjust the temperature to 400 Degrees F and set the timer for 20 minutes. If your garlic head is a bit smaller, check it after 15 minutes
3. When done, garlic should be golden brown and very soft
4. To serve, cloves should pop out and easily be spread or sliced. Store in an airtight container in the refrigerator up to 5 days.
5. You may also freeze individual cloves on a baking sheet, then store together in a freezer-safe storage bag once frozen.

- **Nutrition Info:** Calories: 11; Protein: 2g; Fiber: 1g; Fat: 7g; Carbs: 0g

113.Seven-layer Tostadas

Servings: 6
Cooking Time: 5 Minutes
Ingredients:

- 1 (16-ounce) can refried pinto beans
- 1-1/2 cups guacamole
- 1 cup light sour cream
- 1/2 teaspoon taco seasoning
- 1 cup shredded Mexican cheese blend
- 1 cup chopped tomatoes
- 1/2 cup thinly sliced green onions
- 1/2 cup sliced black olives
- 6-8 whole wheat flour tortillas small enough to fit in your oven
- Olive oil

Directions:

1. Start by placing baking sheet into toaster oven while preheating it to 450°F. Remove pan and drizzle with olive oil.
2. Place tortillas on pan and cook in oven until they are crisp, turn at least once, this should take about 5 minutes or less.
3. In a medium bowl, mash refried beans to break apart any chunks, then microwave for 2 1/2 minutes.
4. Stir taco seasoning into the sour cream. Chop vegetables and halve olives.
5. Top tortillas with ingredients in this order: refried beans, guacamole, sour cream, shredded cheese, tomatoes, onions, and olives.

- **Nutrition Info:** Calories: 657, Sodium: 581 mg, Dietary Fiber: 16.8 g, Total Fat: 31.7 g, Total Carbs: 71.3 g, Protein: 28.9 g.

114.Coriander Artichokes(3)

Servings: 4
Cooking Time: 12 Minutes
Ingredients:

- 12 oz. artichoke hearts
- 1 tbsp. lemon juice
- 1 tsp. coriander, ground
- ½ tsp. cumin seeds
- ½ tsp. olive oil
- Salt and black pepper to taste.

Directions:

1. In a pan that fits your air fryer, mix all the ingredients, toss, introduce the pan in the fryer and cook at 370°F for 15 minutes

2. Divide the mix between plates and serve as a side dish.

- **Nutrition Info:** Calories: 200; Fat: 7g; Fiber: 2g; Carbs: 5g; Protein: 8g

115.Coconut Shrimp With Dip

Servings: 4
Cooking Time: 9 Minutes
Ingredients:

- 1 lb large raw shrimp peeled and deveined with tail on
- 2 eggs beaten
- ¼ cup Panko Breadcrumbs
- 1 tsp salt
- ¼ tsp black pepper
- ½ cup All-Purpose Flour
- ½ cup unsweetened shredded coconut
- Oil for spraying

Directions:

1. Clean and dry the shrimp. Set it aside.
2. Take 3 bowls. Put flour in the first bowl. Beat eggs in the second bowl. Mix coconut, breadcrumbs, salt, and black pepper in the third bowl.
3. Select the Air Fry option and adjust the temperature to 390°F. Push start and preheating will start.
4. Dip each shrimp in flour followed by the egg and then coconut mixture, ensuring shrimp is covered on all sides during each dip.
5. Once the preheating is done, place shrimp in a single layer on greased tray in the basket of the Instant Pot Duo Crisp Air Fryer.
6. Spray the shrimp with oil lightly, and then close the Air Fryer basket lid. Cook for around 4 minutes.
7. After 4 minutes
8. open the Air Fryer basket lid and flip the shrimp over. Respray the shrimp with oil, close the Air Fryer basket lid, and cook for five more minutes.
9. Remove shrimp from the basket and serve with Thai Sweet Chili Sauce.

- **Nutrition Info:** Calories 279, Total Fat 11g, Total Carbs 17g, Protein 28g

116.Amazing Mac And Cheese

Servings:
Cooking Time: 12 Minutes
Ingredients:

- 1 cup cooked macaroni
- 1/2 cup warm milk
- 1 tablespoon parmesan cheese
- 1 cup grated cheddar cheese
- salt and pepper; to taste

Directions:

1. Preheat the Air Fryer to 350 - degrees Fahrenheit. Stir all of the ingredients; except Parmesan, in a baking dish.
2. Place the dish inside the Air Fryer and cook for 10 minutes. Top with the Parmesan cheese.

117.Fried Paprika Tofu

Servings:
Cooking Time: 12 Minutes
Ingredients:

- 1 block extra firm tofu; pressed to remove excess water and cut into cubes
- 1/4 cup cornstarch
- 1 tablespoon smoked paprika
- salt and pepper to taste

Directions:

1. Line the Air Fryer basket with aluminum foil and brush with oil. Preheat the Air Fryer to 370 - degrees Fahrenheit.
2. Mix all ingredients in a bowl. Toss to combine. Place in the Air Fryer basket and cook for 12 minutes.

DINNER RECIPES

118. Lemon Garlic Shrimps

Servings: 2
Cooking Time: 8 Minutes
Ingredients:

- ¾ pound medium shrimp, peeled and deveined
- 1½ tablespoons fresh lemon juice
- 1 tablespoon olive oil
- 1 teaspoon lemon pepper
- ¼ teaspoon paprika
- ¼ teaspoon garlic powder

Directions:

1. Preheat the Air fryer to 400 degree F and grease an Air fryer basket.
2. Mix lemon juice, olive oil, lemon pepper, paprika and garlic powder in a large bowl.
3. Stir in the shrimp and toss until well combined.
4. Arrange shrimp into the Air fryer basket in a single layer and cook for about 8 minutes.
5. Dish out the shrimp in serving plates and serve warm.

- **Nutrition Info:** Calories: 260, Fat: 12.4g, Carbohydrates: 0.3g, Sugar: 0.1g, Protein: 35.6g, Sodium: 619mg

119. Easy Air Fryed Roasted Asparagus

Servings: 4
Cooking Time: 10 Minutes
Ingredients:

- 1 bunch fresh asparagus
- 1 ½ tsp herbs de provence
- Fresh lemon wedge (optional)
- 1 tablespoon olive oil or cooking spray
- Salt and pepper to taste

Directions:

1. Wash asparagus and trim off hard ends
2. Drizzle asparagus with olive oil and add seasonings
3. Place asparagus in air fryer and cook on 360F for 6 to 10 minutes
4. Drizzle squeezed lemon over roasted asparagus.

- **Nutrition Info:** Calories 46 protein 2g fat 3g net carbs 1g

120. One-pan Shrimp And Chorizo Mix Grill

Servings: 4
Cooking Time: 15 Minutes
Ingredients:

- 1 ½ pounds large shrimps, peeled and deveined
- Salt and pepper to taste
- 6 links fresh chorizo sausage
- 2 bunches asparagus spears, trimmed
- Lime wedges

Directions:

1. Place the instant pot air fryer lid on and preheat the instant pot at 390 degrees F.
2. Place the grill pan accessory in the instant pot.
3. Season the shrimps with salt and pepper to taste. Set aside.
4. Place the chorizo on the grill pan and the sausage.
5. Place the asparagus on top.
6. Close the air fryer lid and grill for 15 minutes.
7. Serve with lime wedges.

- **Nutrition Info:** Calories:124 ; Carbs: 9.4g; Protein: 8.2g; Fat: 7.1g

121. Hasselback Potatoes

Servings: 4
Cooking Time: 30 Minutes
Ingredients:

- 4 potatoes
- 2 tablespoons Parmesan cheese, shredded
- 1 tablespoon fresh chives, chopped
- 2 tablespoons olive oil

Directions:

1. Preheat the Air fryer to 355 ºF and grease an Air fryer basket.
2. Cut slits along each potato about ¼-inch apart with a sharp knife, making sure slices should stay connected at the bottom.
3. Coat the potatoes with olive oil and arrange into the Air fryer basket.
4. Cook for about 30 minutes and dish out in a platter.
5. Top with chives and Parmesan cheese to serve.

- **Nutrition Info:** Calories: 218, Fat: 7.9g, Carbohydrates: 33.6g, Sugar: 2.5g, Protein: 4.6g, Sodium: 55mg

122.Garlic Parmesan Shrimp

Servings: 2
Cooking Time: 10 Minutes
Ingredients:

- 1 pound shrimp, deveined and peeled
- ½ cup parmesan cheese, grated
- ¼ cup cilantro, diced
- 1 tablespoon olive oil
- 1 teaspoon salt
- 1 teaspoon fresh cracked pepper
- 1 tablespoon lemon juice
- 6 garlic cloves, diced

Directions:

1. Preheat the Air fryer to 350 degree F and grease an Air fryer basket.
2. Drizzle shrimp with olive oil and lemon juice and season with garlic, salt and cracked pepper.
3. Cover the bowl with plastic wrap and refrigerate for about 3 hours.
4. Stir in the parmesan cheese and cilantro to the bowl and transfer to the Air fryer basket.
5. Cook for about 10 minutes and serve immediately.
- **Nutrition Info:** Calories: 602, Fat: 23.9g, Carbohydrates: 46.5g, Sugar: 2.9g, Protein: 11.3g, Sodium: 886mg

123.Cheesy Shrimp

Servings: 4
Cooking Time: 20 Minutes
Ingredients:

- 2/3 cup Parmesan cheese, grated
- 2 pounds shrimp, peeled and deveined
- 4 garlic cloves, minced
- 2 tablespoons olive oil
- 1 teaspoon dried basil
- ½ teaspoon dried oregano
- 1 teaspoon onion powder
- ½ teaspoon red pepper flakes, crushed
- Ground black pepper, as required
- 2 tablespoons fresh lemon juice

Directions:

1. Preheat the Air fryer to 350 degree F and grease an Air fryer basket.
2. Mix Parmesan cheese, garlic, olive oil, herbs, and spices in a large bowl.
3. Arrange half of the shrimp into the Air fryer basket in a single layer and cook for about 10 minutes.
4. Dish out the shrimps onto serving plates and drizzle with lemon juice to serve hot.
- **Nutrition Info:** Calories: 386, Fat: 14.2g, Carbohydrates: 5.3g, Sugar: 0.4g, Protein: 57.3g, Sodium: 670mg

124.Coconut Crusted Shrimp

Servings: 3
Cooking Time: 40 Minutes
Ingredients:

- 8 ounces coconut milk
- ½ cup sweetened coconut, shredded
- ½ cup panko breadcrumbs
- 1 pound large shrimp, peeled and deveined
- Salt and black pepper, to taste

Directions:

1. Preheat the Air fryer to 350-degree F and grease an Air fryer basket.
2. Place the coconut milk in a shallow bowl.
3. Mix coconut, breadcrumbs, salt, and black pepper in another bowl.
4. Dip each shrimp into coconut milk and finally, dredge in the coconut mixture.
5. Arrange half of the shrimps into the Air fryer basket and cook for about 20 minutes.
6. Dish out the shrimps onto serving plates and repeat with the remaining mixture to serve.
- **Nutrition Info:** Calories: 408, Fats: 23.7g, Carbohydrates: 11.7g, Sugar: 3.4g, Proteins: 31g, Sodium: 253mg

125.Air Fryer Roasted Broccoli

Servings: 4
Cooking Time: 10 Minutes
Ingredients:

- 1 tsp. herbes de provence seasoning (optional)
- 4 cups fresh broccoli
- 1 tablespoon olive oil
- Salt and pepper to taste

Directions:

1. Drizzle or spray broccoli with olive and sprinkle seasoning throughout
2. Spray air fryer basket with cooking oil, place broccoli and cook for 5-8 minutes on 360F
3. Open air fryer and examine broccoli after 5 minutes because different fryer brands cook at different rates.
- **Nutrition Info:** Calories 61 Fat 4g protein 3g net carbs 4g

126.Rich Meatloaf With Mustard And Peppers

Servings: 5
Cooking Time: 20 Minutes
Ingredients:

- 1 pound beef, ground
- 1/2 pound veal, ground
- 1 egg
- 4 tablespoons vegetable juice
- 1/2 cup pork rinds
- 2 bell peppers, chopped
- 1 onion, chopped
- 2 garlic cloves, minced
- 2 tablespoons tomato paste
- 2 tablespoons soy sauce
- 1 (1-ouncepackage ranch dressing mix
- Sea salt, to taste
- 1/2 teaspoon ground black pepper, to taste
- 7 ounces tomato puree
- 1 tablespoon Dijon mustard

Directions:

1. Start by preheating your Air Fryer to 330 degrees F.
2. In a mixing bowl, thoroughly combine the ground beef, veal, egg, vegetable juice, pork rinds, bell peppers, onion, garlic, tomato paste, soy sauce, ranch dressing mix, salt, and ground black pepper.
3. Mix until everything is well incorporated and press into a lightly greased meatloaf pan.
4. Cook approximately 25 minutes in the preheated Air Fryer. Whisk the tomato puree with the mustard and spread the topping over the top of your meatloaf.

5. Continue to cook 2 minutes more. Let it stand on a cooling rack for 6 minutes before slicing and serving. Enjoy!
- **Nutrition Info:** 398 Calories; 24g Fat; 9g Carbs; 32g Protein; 3g Sugars; 6g Fiber

127.Green Beans And Mushroom Casserole

Servings: 6
Cooking Time: 12 Minutes
Ingredients:

- 24 ounces fresh green beans, trimmed
- 2 cups fresh button mushrooms, sliced
- 1/3 cup French fried onions
- 3 tablespoons olive oil
- 2 tablespoons fresh lemon juice
- 1 teaspoon ground sage
- 1 teaspoon garlic powder
- 1 teaspoon onion powder
- Salt and black pepper, to taste

Directions:

1. Preheat the Air fryer to 400 ºF and grease an Air fryer basket.
2. Mix the green beans, mushrooms, oil, lemon juice, sage, and spices in a bowl and toss to coat well.
3. Arrange the green beans mixture into the Air fryer basket and cook for about 12 minutes.
4. Dish out in a serving dish and top with fried onions to serve.
- **Nutrition Info:** Calories: 65, Fat: 1.6g, Carbohydrates: 11g, Sugar: 2.4g, Protein: 3g, Sodium: 52mg

128.Easy Marinated London Broil

Servings: 4
Cooking Time: 20 Minutes
Ingredients:

- For the marinade:
- 2 tablespoons Worcestershire sauce
- 2 garlic cloves, minced
- 1 tablespoon oil
- 2 tablespoons rice vinegar
- London Broil:
- 2 pounds London broil
- 2 tablespoons tomato paste
- Sea salt and cracked black pepper, to taste

- 1 tablespoon mustard

Directions:
1. Combine all the marinade ingredients in a mixing bowl; add the London boil to the bowl. Cover and let it marinate for 3 hours.
2. Preheat the Air Fryer to 400 degrees F. Spritz the Air Fryer grill pan with cooking oil.
3. Grill the marinated London broil in the preheated Air Fryer for 18 minutes. Turn London broil over, top with the tomato paste, salt, black pepper, and mustard.
4. Continue to grill an additional 10 minutes. Serve immediately.
- **Nutrition Info:** 517 Calories; 21g Fat; 5g Carbs; 70g Protein; 4g Sugars; 7g Fiber

129.Green Beans And Lime Sauce

Servings: 4
Cooking Time: 20 Minutes
Ingredients:
- 1 lb. green beans, trimmed
- 2 tbsp. ghee; melted
- 1 tbsp. lime juice
- 1 tsp. chili powder
- A pinch of salt and black pepper

Directions:
1. Take a bowl and mix the ghee with the rest of the ingredients except the green beans and whisk really well.
2. Mix the green beans with the lime sauce, toss
3. Put them in your air fryer's basket and cook at 400°F for 8 minutes. Serve right away.
- **Nutrition Info:** Calories: 151; Fat: 4g; Fiber: 2g; Carbs: 4g; Protein: 6g

130.Stuffed Okra

Servings: 2
Cooking Time: 12 Minutes
Ingredients:
- 8 ounces large okra
- ¼ cup chickpea flour
- ¼ of onion, chopped
- 2 tablespoons coconut, grated freshly
- 1 teaspoon garam masala powder
- ½ teaspoon ground turmeric
- ½ teaspoon red chili powder

- ½ teaspoon ground cumin
- Salt, to taste

Directions:
1. Preheat the Air fryer to 390 ºF and grease an Air fryer basket.
2. Mix the flour, onion, grated coconut, and spices in a bowl and toss to coat well.
3. Stuff the flour mixture into okra and arrange into the Air fryer basket.
4. Cook for about 12 minutes and dish out in a serving plate.
- **Nutrition Info:** Calories: 166, Fat: 3.7g, Carbohydrates: 26.6g, Sugar: 5.3g, Protein: 7.6g, Sodium: 103mg

131.Cheese Breaded Pork

Servings: 6
Cooking Time: 15 Minutes
Ingredients:
- 6 pork chops
- 6 tbsp seasoned breadcrumbs
- 2 tbsp parmesan cheese, grated
- 1 tbsp melted butter
- ½ cup mozzarella cheese, shredded
- 1 tbsp marinara sauce

Directions:
1. Preheat your air fryer to 390 f. Grease the cooking basket with cooking spray. In a small bowl, mix breadcrumbs and parmesan cheese. In another microwave proof bowl, add butter and melt in the microwave.
2. Brush the pork with butter and dredge into the breadcrumbs. Add pork to the cooking basket and cook for 6 minutes. Turnover and top with marinara sauce and shredded mozzarella; cook for 3 more minutes
- **Nutrition Info:** Calories: 431 Cal Total Fat: 0 g Saturated Fat: 0 g Cholesterol: 0 mg Sodium: 0 mg Total Carbs: 0 g Fiber: 0 g Sugar: 0 g Protein: 0 g

132.Grilled Halibut With Tomatoes And Hearts Of Palm

Servings: 4
Cooking Time: 15 Minutes
Ingredients:
- 4 halibut fillets

- Juice from 1 lemon
- Salt and pepper to taste
- 2 tablespoons oil
- ½ cup hearts of palm, rinse and drained
- 1 cup cherry tomatoes

Directions:
1. Place the instant pot air fryer lid on and preheat the instant pot at 390 degrees F.
2. Place the grill pan accessory in the instant pot.
3. Season the halibut fillets with lemon juice, salt, and pepper. Brush with oil.
4. Place the fish on the grill pan.
5. Arrange the hearts of palms and cherry tomatoes on the side and sprinkle with more salt and pepper.
6. Close the air fryer lid and cook for 15 minutes.
- **Nutrition Info:** Calories: 208; Carbs: 7g; Protein: 21 g; Fat: 11g

133. Roasted Butternut Squash With Brussels Sprouts & Sweet Potato Noodles

Servings: 2
Cooking Time: 15 Minutes
Ingredients:
- Squash:
- 3 cups chopped butternut squash
- 2 teaspoons extra light olive oil
- 1/8 teaspoon sea salt
- Veggies:
- 5-6 Brussels sprouts
- 5 fresh shiitake mushrooms
- 2 cloves garlic
- 1/2 teaspoon black sesame seeds
- 1/2 teaspoon white sesame seeds
- A few sprinkles ground pepper
- A small pinch red pepper flakes
- 1 tablespoon extra light olive oil
- 1 teaspoon sesame oil
- 1 teaspoon onion powder
- 1 teaspoon garlic powder
- 1/4 teaspoon sea salt
- Noodles:
- 1 bundle sweet potato vermicelli
- 2-3 teaspoons low-sodium soy sauce

Directions:
1. Start by soaking potato vermicelli in water for at least 2 hours.
2. Preheat toaster oven to 375°F.
3. Place squash on a baking sheet with edges, then drizzle with olive oil and sprinkle with salt and pepper. Mix together well on pan.
4. Bake the squash for 30 minutes, mixing and flipping half way through.
5. Remove the stems from the mushrooms and chop the Brussels sprouts.
6. Chop garlic and mix the veggies.
7. Drizzle sesame and olive oil over the mixture, then add garlic powder, onion powder, sesame seeds, red pepper flakes, salt, and pepper.
8. Bake veggie mix for 15 minutes.
9. While the veggies bake, put noodles in a small sauce pan and add just enough water to cover.
10. Bring water to a rolling boil and boil noodles for about 8 minutes.
11. Drain noodles and combine with squash and veggies in a large bowl.
12. Drizzle with soy sauce, sprinkle with sesame seeds, and serve.
- **Nutrition Info:** Calories: 409, Sodium: 1124 mg, Dietary Fiber: 12.2 g, Total Fat: 15.6 g, Total Carbs: 69.3 g, Protein: 8.8 g.

134. Sage Sausages Balls

Servings: 4
Cooking Time: 20 Minutes
Ingredients:
- 3 ½ oz sausages, sliced
- Salt and black pepper to taste
- 1 cup onion, chopped
- 3 tbsp breadcrumbs
- ½ tsp garlic puree
- 1 tsp sage

Directions:
1. Preheat your air fryer to 340 f. In a bowl, mix onions, sausage meat, sage, garlic puree, salt and pepper. Add breadcrumbs to a plate. Form balls using the mixture and roll them in breadcrumbs. Add onion balls in your air fryer's cooking basket and cook for 15 minutes. Serve and enjoy!

- **Nutrition Info:** Calories: 162 Cal Total Fat: 12.1 g Saturated Fat: 0 g Cholesterol: 25 mg Sodium: 324 mg Total Carbs: 7.3 g Fiber: 0 g Sugar: 0 g Protein: 6 g

135.Rice And Tuna Puff

Servings: 6
Cooking Time: 60 Minutes
Ingredients:

- 2/3 cup uncooked white rice
- 1 1/3 cups water
- 1/3 cup butter
- 1/4 cup all-purpose flour
- 1 teaspoon salt
- 1/4 teaspoon ground black pepper
- 1 1/2 cups milk
- 2 egg yolks
- 1 (12 ounces) can tuna, undrained
- 2 tablespoons grated onion
- 1 tablespoon lemon juice
- 2 egg whites

Directions:

1. In a saucepan, bring water to a boil. Stir in rice, cover, and cook on low heat until liquid is fully absorbed, around 20 minutes.
2. In another saucepan over medium heat, melt butter. Stir in pepper, salt, and flour. Cook for 2 minutes, whisking constantly and slowly adding milk. Continue cooking and stirring until thickened.
3. In a medium bowl, whisk egg yolks. Slowly whisk in half of the thickened milk mixture. Add to a pan of remaining milk and continue cooking and stirring for 2 more minutes. Stir in lemon juice, onion, tuna, and rice.
4. Place the instant pot air fryer lid on, lightly grease baking pan of the instant pot with cooking spray. And transfer rice mixture into it.
5. Beat egg whites until stiff peak forms. Slowly fold into rice mixture.
6. Cover pan with foil, place the baking pan in the instant pot and close the air fryer lid.
7. Cook at 360 ºF for 20 minutes.
8. Cook for 15 minutes at 390 ºF until tops are lightly browned and the middle has set.
9. Serve and enjoy.

- **Nutrition Info:** Calories: 302; Carbs: 24.1g; Protein: 20.6g; Fat: 13.6g

136.Bbq Pork Ribs

Servings: 2 To 3
Cooking Time: 5 Hrs 30 Minutes
Ingredients:

- 1 lb pork ribs
- 1 tsp soy sauce
- Salt and black pepper to taste
- 1 tsp oregano
- 1 tbsp + 1 tbsp maple syrup
- 3 tbsp barbecue sauce
- 2 cloves garlic, minced
- 1 tbsp cayenne pepper
- 1 tsp sesame oil

Directions:

1. Put the chops on a chopping board and use a knife to cut them into smaller pieces of desired sizes. Put them in a mixing bowl, add the soy sauce, salt, pepper, oregano, one tablespoon of maple syrup, barbecue sauce, garlic, cayenne pepper, and sesame oil. Mix well and place the pork in the fridge to marinate in the spices for 5 hours.
2. Preheat the Air Fryer to 350 F. Open the Air Fryer and place the ribs in the fryer basket. Slide the fryer basket in and cook for 15 minutes. Open the Air fryer, turn the ribs using tongs, apply the remaining maple syrup with a brush, close the Air Fryer, and continue cooking for 10 minutes.

- **Nutrition Info:** 346 Calories; 11g Fat; 4g Carbs; 32g Protein; 1g Sugars; 1g Fiber

137.Tex-mex Chicken Quesadillas

Servings: 4
Cooking Time: 10 Minutes
Ingredients:

- 2 green onions
- 2 cups shredded skinless rotisserie chicken meat
- 1-1/2 cups shredded Monterey Jack cheese
- 1 pickled jalapeño
- 1/4 cup fresh cilantro leaves
- 4 burrito-size flour tortillas
- 1/2 cup reduced-fat sour cream

Directions:

1. Start by preheating toaster oven to 425°F.
2. Thinly slice the green onions and break apart.
3. Mix together chicken, cheese, jalapeño, and onions in a bowl, then evenly divide mixture onto one half of each tortilla.
4. Fold opposite half over mixture and place quesadillas onto a baking sheet.
5. Bake for 10 minutes.
6. Cut in halves or quarters and serve with sour cream.
- **Nutrition Info:** Calories: 830, Sodium: 921 mg, Dietary Fiber: 1.8 g, Total Fat: 59.0 g, Total Carbs: 13.8 g, Protein: 60.8 g.

138.Fish Cakes With Horseradish Sauce

Servings: 4
Cooking Time: 20 Minutes
Ingredients:
- Halibut Cakes:
- 1 pound halibut
- 2 tablespoons olive oil
- 1/2 teaspoon cayenne pepper
- 1/4 teaspoon black pepper
- Salt, to taste
- 2 tablespoons cilantro, chopped
- 1 shallot, chopped
- 2 garlic cloves, minced
- 1 cup Romano cheese, grated
- 1 egg, whisked
- 1 tablespoon Worcestershire sauce
- Mayo Sauce:
- 1 teaspoon horseradish, grated
- 1/2 cup mayonnaise

Directions:
1. Start by preheating your Air Fryer to 380 degrees F. Spritz the Air Fryer basket with cooking oil.
2. Mix all ingredients for the halibut cakes in a bowl; knead with your hands until everything is well incorporated.
3. Shape the mixture into equally sized patties. Transfer your patties to the Air Fryer basket. Cook the fish patties for 10 minutes, turning them over halfway through.
4. Mix the horseradish and mayonnaise. Serve the halibut cakes with the horseradish mayo.

- **Nutrition Info:** 532 Calories; 32g Fat; 3g Carbs; 28g Protein; 3g Sugars; 6g Fiber

139.Coconut-crusted Haddock With Curried Pumpkin Seeds

Servings: 4
Cooking Time: 10 Minutes
Ingredients:
- 2 teaspoons canola oil
- 2 teaspoons honey
- 1 teaspoon curry powder
- 1/4 teaspoon ground cinnamon
- 1 teaspoon salt
- 1 cup pumpkin seeds
- 1-1/2 pounds haddock or cod filets
- 1/2 cup roughly grated unsweetened coconut
- 3/4 cups panko-style bread crumbs
- 2 tablespoons butter, melted
- 3 tablespoons apricot fruit spread
- 1 tablespoon lime juice

Directions:
1. Start by preheating toaster oven to 350°F.
2. In a medium bowl, mix honey, oil, curry powder, 1/2 teaspoon salt, and cinnamon.
3. Add pumpkin seeds to the bowl and toss to coat, then lay flat on a baking sheet.
4. Toast for 14 minutes, then transfer to a bowl to cool.
5. Increase the oven temperature to 450°F.
6. Brush a baking sheet with oil and lay filets flat.
7. In another medium mixing bowl, mix together bread crumbs, butter, and remaining salt.
8. In a small bowl mash together apricot spread and lime juice.
9. Brush each filet with apricot mixture, then press bread crumb mixture onto each piece.
10. Bake for 10 minutes.
11. Transfer to a plate and top with pumpkin seeds to serve.
- **Nutrition Info:** Calories: 273, Sodium: 491 mg, Dietary Fiber: 6.1 g, Total Fat: 8.4 g, Total Carbs: 47.3 g, Protein: 7.0 g.

140.Creole Beef Meatloaf

Servings: 6

Cooking Time: 15 Minutes

Ingredients:

- 1 lb. ground beef
- 1/2 tablespoon butter
- 1 red bell pepper diced
- 1/3 cup red onion diced
- 1/3 cup cilantro diced
- 1/3 cup zucchini diced
- 1 tablespoon creole seasoning
- 1/2 teaspoon turmeric
- 1/2 teaspoon cumin
- 1/2 teaspoon coriander
- 2 garlic cloves minced
- Salt and black pepper to taste

Directions:

1. Mix the beef minced with all the meatball ingredients in a bowl.
2. Make small meatballs out of this mixture and place them in the Air fryer basket.
3. Press "Power Button" of Air Fry Oven and turn the dial to select the "Air Fry" mode.
4. Press the Time button and again turn the dial to set the cooking time to 15 minutes.
5. Now push the Temp button and rotate the dial to set the temperature at 370 degrees F.
6. Once preheated, place the Air fryer basket in the oven and close its lid.
7. Slice and serve warm.
- **Nutrition Info:** Calories: 331 Cal Total Fat: 2.5 g Saturated Fat: 0.5 g Cholesterol: 35 mg Sodium: 595 mg Total Carbs: 69 g Fiber: 12.2 g Sugar: 12.5 g Protein: 26.7 g

141.Pesto & White Wine Salmon

Servings: 4
Cooking Time: 10 Minutes

Ingredients:

- 1-1/4 pounds salmon filet
- 2 tablespoons white wine
- 2 tablespoons pesto
- 1 lemon

Directions:

1. Cut the salmon into 4 pieces and place on a greased baking sheet.
2. Slice the lemon into quarters and squeeze 1 quarter over each piece of salmon.

3. Drizzle wine over salmon and set aside to marinate while preheating the toaster oven on broil.
4. Spread pesto over each piece of salmon.
5. Broil for at least 10 minutes, or until the fish is cooked to desired doneness and the pesto is browned.
- **Nutrition Info:** Calories: 236, Sodium: 111 mg, Dietary Fiber: 0.9 g, Total Fat: 12.1 g, Total Carbs: 3.3 g, Protein: 28.6 g.

142.Zingy Dilled Salmon

Servings: 2
Cooking Time: 20 Minutes

Ingredients:

- 2 salmon steaks
- Coarse sea salt, to taste
- 1/4 teaspoon freshly ground black pepper, or more to taste
- 1 tablespoon sesame oil
- Zest of 1 lemon
- 1 tablespoon fresh lemon juice
- 1 teaspoon garlic, minced
- 1/2 teaspoon smoked cayenne pepper
- 1/2 teaspoon dried dill

Directions:

1. Preheat your Air Fryer to 380 degrees F. Pat dry the salmon steaks with a kitchen towel.
2. In a ceramic dish, combine the remaining ingredients until everything is well whisked.
3. Add the salmon steaks to the ceramic dish and let them sit in the refrigerator for 1 hour. Now, place the salmon steaks in the cooking basket. Reserve the marinade.
4. Cook for 12 minutes, flipping halfway through the cooking time.
5. Meanwhile, cook the marinade in a small sauté pan over a moderate flame. Cook until the sauce has thickened.
6. Pour the sauce over the steaks and serve.
- **Nutrition Info:** 476 Calories; 18g Fat; 2g Carbs; 47g Protein; 8g Sugars; 4g Fiber

143.Party Stuffed Pork Chops

Servings: 4
Cooking Time: 40 Minutes

Ingredients:

- 8 pork chops

- ¼ tsp pepper
- 4 cups stuffing mix
- ½ tsp salt
- 2 tbsp olive oil
- 4 garlic cloves, minced
- 2 tbsp sage leaves

Directions:

1. Preheat your air fryer to 350 f. cut a hole in pork chops and fill chops with stuffing mix. In a bowl, mix sage leaves, garlic cloves, oil, salt and pepper. Cover chops with marinade and let marinate for 10 minutes. Place the chops in your air fryer's cooking basket and cook for 25 minutes. Serve and enjoy!
- **Nutrition Info:** Calories: 364 Cal Total Fat: 13 g Saturated Fat: 4 g Cholesterol: 119 mg Sodium: 349 mg Total Carbs: 19 g Fiber: 3 g Sugar: 6 g Protein: 40 g

144.Mozzarella & Olive Pizza Bagels

Servings: 4
Cooking Time: 10 Minutes
Ingredients:
- 2 whole wheat bagels
- 1/4 cup marinara sauce
- 1/4 teaspoon Italian seasoning
- 1/8 teaspoon red pepper flakes
- 3/4 cup shredded low-moisture mozzarella cheese
- 1/4 cup chopped green pepper
- 3 tablespoons sliced black olives
- Fresh basil
- 1 teaspoon parmesan cheese

Directions:

1. Start by preheating toaster oven to 375°F and lining a pan with parchment paper.
2. Cut bagels in half and lay on pan with inside facing up. Spread sauce over each half.
3. Sprinkle red pepper flakes and 2 tablespoons of mozzarella over each half.
4. Top each half with olives and peppers and then top with another tablespoon of mozzarella.
5. Bake for 8 minutes, then switch to broil setting and broil for another 2 minutes. Top with basil and parmesan and serve.

- **Nutrition Info:** Calories: 222, Sodium: 493 mg, Dietary Fiber: 1.9 g, Total Fat: 6.1 g, Total Carbs: 30.2 g, Protein: 12.1 g.

145.Venetian Liver

Servings: 6
Cooking Time: 15-30;
Ingredients:
- 500g veal liver
- 2 white onions
- 100g of water
- 2 tbsp vinegar
- Salt and pepper to taste

Directions:

1. Chop the onion and put it inside the pan with the water. Set the air fryer to 1800C and cook for 20 minutes.
2. Add the liver cut into small pieces and vinegar, close the lid, and cook for an additional 10 minutes.
3. Add salt and pepper.
- **Nutrition Info:** Calories 131, Fat 14.19 g, Carbohydrates 16.40 g, Sugars 5.15 g, Protein 25.39 g, Cholesterol 350.41 mg

146.Flank Steak Beef

Servings: 4
Cooking Time: 20 Minutes
Ingredients:
- 1 pound flank steaks, sliced
- ¼ cup xanthum gum
- 2 teaspoon vegetable oil
- ½ teaspoon ginger
- ½ cup soy sauce
- 1 tablespoon garlic, minced
- ½ cup water
- ¾ cup swerve, packed

Directions:

1. Preheat the Air fryer to 390 degree F and grease an Air fryer basket.
2. Coat the steaks with xanthum gum on both the sides and transfer into the Air fryer basket.
3. Cook for about 10 minutes and dish out in a platter.
4. Meanwhile, cook rest of the ingredients for the sauce in a saucepan.

5. Bring to a boil and pour over the steak slices to serve.
- **Nutrition Info:** Calories: 372, Fat: 11.8g, Carbohydrates: 1.8g, Sugar: 27.3g, Protein: 34g, Sodium: 871mg

147.Cheese And Garlic Stuffed Chicken Breasts

Servings: 2
Cooking Time: 20 Minutes
Ingredients:
- 1/2 cup Cottage cheese 2 eggs, beaten
- 2 medium-sized chicken breasts, halved
- 2 tablespoons fresh coriander, chopped 1tsp. fine sea salt
- Seasoned breadcrumbs
- 1/3 tsp. freshly ground black pepper, to savor 3 cloves garlic, finely minced

Directions:
1. Firstly, flatten out the chicken breast using a meat tenderizer.
2. In a medium-sized mixing dish, combine the Cottage cheese with the garlic, coriander, salt, and black pepper.
3. Spread 1/3 of the mixture over the first chicken breast. Repeat with the remaining ingredients. Roll the chicken around the filling; make sure to secure with toothpicks.
4. Now, whisk the egg in a shallow bowl. In another shallow bowl, combine the salt, ground black pepper, and seasoned breadcrumbs.
5. Coat the chicken breasts with the whisked egg; now, roll them in the breadcrumbs.
6. Cook in the air fryer cooking basket at 365 °F for 22 minutes. Serve immediately.
- **Nutrition Info:** 424 Calories; 24.5g Fat; 7.5g Carbs; 43.4g Protein; 5.3g Sugars

148.Coco Mug Cake

Servings: 1
Cooking Time: 20 Minutes
Ingredients:
- 1 large egg.
- 2 tbsp. granular erythritol.
- 2 tbsp. coconut flour.
- 2 tbsp. heavy whipping cream.
- ¼ tsp. baking powder.

- ¼ tsp. vanilla extract.

Directions:
1. In a 4-inch ramekin, whisk egg, then add remaining ingredients. Stir until smooth. Place into the air fryer basket.
2. Adjust the temperature to 300 Degrees F and set the timer for 25 minutes.
3. When done a toothpick should come out clean. Enjoy right out of the ramekin with a spoon. Serve warm.
- **Nutrition Info:** Calories: 237; Protein: 9g; Fiber: 0g; Fat: 14g; Carbs: 47g

149.Cajun Fish Fritters

Servings: 4
Cooking Time: 20 Minutes
Ingredients:
- 2 catfish fillets
- 1 cup parmesan cheese
- 3 ounces butter
- 1 teaspoon baking powder
- 1 teaspoon baking soda
- 1/2 cup buttermilk
- 1 teaspoon Cajun seasoning
- 1 cup Swiss cheese, shredded

Directions:
1. Bring a pot of salted water to a boil. Boil the fish fillets for 5 minutes or until it is opaque. Flake the fish into small pieces.
2. Mix the remaining ingredients in a bowl; add the fish and mix until well combined. Shape the fish mixture into 12 patties.
3. Cook in the preheated Air Fryer at 380 degrees F for 15 minutes. Work in batches. Enjoy!
- **Nutrition Info:** 478 Calories; 31g Fat; 22g Carbs; 28g Protein; 2g Sugars; 1g Fiber

150.Lamb Skewers

Servings: 4
Cooking Time: 20 Minutes
Ingredients:
- 2 lb. lamb meat; cubed
- 2 red bell peppers; cut into medium pieces
- ¼ cup olive oil
- 2 tbsp. lemon juice
- 1 tbsp. oregano; dried
- 1 tbsp. red vinegar

- 1 tbsp. garlic; minced
- ½ tsp. rosemary; dried
- A pinch of salt and black pepper

Directions:
1. Take a bowl and mix all the ingredients and toss them well.
2. Thread the lamb and bell peppers on skewers, place them in your air fryer's basket and cook at 380°F for 10 minutes on each side. Divide between plates and serve with a side salad
- **Nutrition Info:** Calories: 274; Fat: 12g; Fiber: 3g; Carbs: 6g; Protein: 16g

151.Stuffed Potatoes

Servings: 4
Cooking Time: 31 Minutes
Ingredients:
- 4 potatoes, peeled
- 1 tablespoon butter
- ½ of brown onion, chopped
- 2 tablespoons chives, chopped
- ½ cup Parmesan cheese, grated
- 3 tablespoons canola oil

Directions:
1. Preheat the Air fryer to 390 ºF and grease an Air fryer basket.
2. Coat the potatoes with canola oil and arrange into the Air fryer basket.
3. Cook for about 20 minutes and transfer into a platter.
4. Cut each potato in half and scoop out the flesh from each half.
5. Heat butter in a frying pan over medium heat and add onions.
6. Sauté for about 5 minutes and dish out in a bowl.
7. Mix the onions with the potato flesh, chives, and half of cheese.
8. Stir well and stuff the potato halves evenly with the onion potato mixture.
9. Top with the remaining cheese and arrange the potato halves into the Air fryer basket.
10. Cook for about 6 minutes and dish out to serve warm.
- **Nutrition Info:** Calories: 328, Fat: 11.3g, Carbohydrates: 34.8g, Sugar: 3.1g, Protein: 5.8g, Sodium: 77mg

152.Vegetable Cane

Servings: 4
Cooking Time: More Than 60 Minutes;
Ingredients:
- 2 calf legs
- 4 carrots
- 4 medium potatoes
- 1 clove garlic
- 300ml Broth
- Leave to taste
- Pepper to taste

Directions:
1. Place the ears, garlic, and half of the broth in the greased basket.
2. Set the temperature to 1800C.
3. Cook the stems for 40 minutes, turning them in the middle of cooking.
4. Add the vegetables in pieces, salt, pepper, pour the rest of the broth and cook for another 50 minutes (time may vary depending on the size of the hocks).
5. Mix the vegetables and the ears 2 to 3 times during cooking.
- **Nutrition Info:** Calories 7.9, Fat 0.49g, Carbohydrate 0.77g, Sugar 0.49g, Protein 0.08mg, Cholesterol 0mg

153.Miso-glazed Salmon

Servings: 4
Cooking Time: 5 Minutes
Ingredients:
- 1/4 cup red or white miso
- 1/3 cup sake
- 1 tablespoon soy sauce
- 2 tablespoons vegetable oil
- 1/4 cup sugar
- 4 skinless salmon filets

Directions:
1. In a shallow bowl, mix together the miso, sake, oil, soy sauce, and sugar.
2. Toss the salmon in the mixture until thoroughly coated on all sides.
3. Preheat your toaster oven to "high" on broil mode.
4. Place salmon in a broiling pan and broil until the top is well charred—about 5 minutes.

- **Nutrition Info:** Calories: 401, Sodium: 315 mg, Dietary Fiber: 0 g, Total Fat: 19.2 g, Total Carbs: 14.1 g, Protein: 39.2 g.

154.Cheese Zucchini Boats

Servings: 2
Cooking Time: 20 Minutes
Ingredients:
- 2 medium zucchinis
- ¼ cup full-fat ricotta cheese
- ¼ cup shredded mozzarella cheese
- ¼ cup low-carb, no-sugar-added pasta sauce.
- 2 tbsp. grated vegetarian Parmesan cheese
- 1 tbsp. avocado oil
- ¼ tsp. garlic powder.
- ½ tsp. dried parsley.
- ¼ tsp. dried oregano.

Directions:
1. Cut off 1-inch from the top and bottom of each zucchini.
2. Slice zucchini in half lengthwise and use a spoon to scoop out a bit of the inside, making room for filling. Brush with oil and spoon 2 tbsp. pasta sauce into each shell
3. Take a medium bowl, mix ricotta, mozzarella, oregano, garlic powder and parsley
4. Spoon the mixture into each zucchini shell. Place stuffed zucchini shells into the air fryer basket.
5. Adjust the temperature to 350 Degrees F and set the timer for 20 minutes
6. To remove from the fryer basket, use tongs or a spatula and carefully lift out. Top with Parmesan. Serve immediately.
- **Nutrition Info:** Calories: 215; Protein: 15g; Fiber: 7g; Fat: 19g; Carbs: 3g

155.Smoked Sausage And Bacon Shashlik

Servings: 4
Cooking Time: 20 Minutes
Ingredients:
- 1 pound smoked Polish beef sausage, sliced

- 1 tablespoon mustard
- 1 tablespoon olive oil
- 2 tablespoons Worcestershire sauce
- 2 bell peppers, sliced
- Salt and ground black pepper, to taste

Directions:
1. Toss the sausage with the mustard, olive, and Worcestershire sauce. Thread sausage and peppers onto skewers.
2. Sprinkle with salt and black pepper.
3. Cook in the preheated Air Fryer at 360 degrees Ffor 11 minutes. Brush the skewers with the reserved marinade.
- **Nutrition Info:** 422 Calories; 36g Fat; 9g Carbs; 18g Protein; 6g Sugars; 7g Fiber

156.Shrimp Scampi

Servings: 6
Cooking Time: 7 Minutes
Ingredients:
- 4 tablespoons salted butter
- 1 pound shrimp, peeled and deveined
- 2 tablespoons fresh basil, chopped
- 1 tablespoon fresh chives, chopped
- 1 tablespoon fresh lemon juice
- 1 tablespoon garlic, minced
- 2 teaspoons red pepper flakes, crushed
- 2 tablespoons dry white wine

Directions:
1. Preheat the Air fryer to 325 ºF and grease an Air fryer pan.
2. Heat butter, lemon juice, garlic, and red pepper flakes in a pan and return the pan to Air fryer basket.
3. Cook for about 2 minutes and stir in shrimp, basil, chives and wine.
4. Cook for about 5 minutes and dish out the mixture onto serving plates.
5. Serve hot.
- **Nutrition Info:** Calories: 250, Fat: 13.7g, Carbohydrates: 3.3g, Sugar: 0.3g, Protein: 26.3g, Sodium: 360mg

MEAT RECIPES

157. Simple Chicken Nuggets

Servings: 4
Cooking Time: 8 Minutes
Ingredients:
- 1 pound (454 g) boneless, skinless chicken breasts, cut into 1-inch pieces
- 2 tablespoons panko bread crumbs
- 6 tablespoons bread crumbs
- Chicken seasoning or rub, to taste
- Salt and ground black pepper, to taste
- 2 eggs
- Cooking spray

Directions:
1. Spritz the air fryer basket with cooking spray.
2. Combine the bread crumbs, chicken seasoning, salt, and black pepper in a large bowl. Stir to mix well. Whisk the eggs in a separate bowl.
3. Dunk the chicken pieces in the egg mixture, then in the breadcrumb mixture. Shake the excess off.
4. Arrange the well-coated chicken pieces in the basket. Spritz with cooking spray.
5. Put the air fryer basket on the baking pan and slide into Rack Position 2, select Air Fry, set temperature to 400ºF (205ºC) and set time to 8 minutes.
6. Flip the chicken halfway through.
7. When cooking is complete, the chicken should be crispy and golden brown.
8. Serve immediately.

158. Sweet & Spicy Chicken

Servings: 6
Cooking Time: 30 Minutes
Ingredients:
- 6 chicken breasts, skinless, boneless, cut in 1-inch pieces
- 1 cup corn starch
- 2 cups water
- 1 cup ketchup
- ½ cup brown sugar
- 1 tbsp. sesame oil
- 3 tbsp. soy sauce
- 2 tbsp. black sesame seeds
- 2 tbsp. white sesame seeds
- ½ tsp red pepper flakes
- ½ tsp garlic powder
- 2 tbsp. green onion, chopped

Directions:
1. Place baking pan in position 2. Lightly spray fryer basket with cooking spray.
2. Place the cornstarch in a large bowl. Add chicken and toss to coat chicken thoroughly.
3. Working in batches, place chicken in a single layer in the basket and place on baking pan. Set oven to air fryer on 350°F for 10 minutes. Stir the chicken halfway through cooking time. Transfer chicken to baking sheet.
4. In a large skillet over medium heat, whisk together remaining ingredients, except green onion. Bring to a boil, stirring occasionally. Cook until sauce has thickened, about 3-5 minutes.
5. Add chicken and stir to coat. Cook another 3-5 minutes, stirring frequently. Serve garnished with green onions.
- **Nutrition Info:** Calories 556, Total Fat 12g, Saturated Fat 3g, Total Carbs 50g, Net Carbs 49g, Protein 62g, Sugar 26g, Fiber 1g, Sodium 730mg, Potassium 957mg, Phosphorus 569mg

159. Savory Chicken With Onion

Servings: 4
Cooking Time: 20 Minutes
Ingredients:
- 4 chicken breasts, cubed
- 1 ½ cup onion soup mix
- 1 cup mushroom soup
- ½ cup heavy cream

Directions:
1. Preheat your Breville Smart oven to 400 F on Bake function. Add mushrooms, onion mix, and heavy cream in a frying pan. Heat on low heat for 1 minute. Pour the warm mixture over chicken and allow to sit for 25 minutes. Place the marinated chicken in the basket and fit in the baking tray; cook for 15 minutes. Serve and enjoy!

160. Minced Venison Grandma's Easy To Cook Wontons With Garlic Paste

Servings:x
Cooking Time:x
Ingredients:

- 1 ½ cup all-purpose flour
- ½ tsp. salt
- 2 tsp. soya sauce
- 5 tbsp. water
- 2 cups minced venison
- 2 tbsp. oil
- 2 tsp. ginger-garlic paste
- 2 tsp. vinegar

Directions:

1. Squeeze the dough and cover it with plastic wrap and set aside. Next, cook the ingredients for the filling and try to ensure that the venison is covered well with the sauce. Roll the dough and place the filling in the center.
2. Now, wrap the dough to cover the filling and pinch the edges together. Pre heat the Breville smart oven at 200° F for 5 minutes.
3. Place the wontons in the fry basket and close it. Let them cook at the same temperature for another 20 minutes. Recommended sides are chili sauce or ketchup.

161. Clams French Cuisine Galette

Servings:x
Cooking Time:x
Ingredients:

- 2 tbsp. garam masala
- 1 lb. minced clam
- 3 tsp ginger finely chopped
- 1-2 tbsp. fresh coriander leaves
- 2 or 3 green chilies finely chopped
- 1 ½ tbsp. lemon juice
- Salt and pepper to taste

Directions:

1. Mix the ingredients in a clean bowl. Mold this mixture into round and flat French Cuisine Galettes. Wet the French Cuisine Galettes slightly with water.
2. Pre heat the Breville smart oven at 160 degrees Fahrenheit for 5 minutes. Place the French Cuisine Galettes in the fry basket and let them cook for another 25 minutes at the same temperature.
3. Keep rolling them over to get a uniform cook. Serve either with mint sauce or ketchup.

162. Tasty Lemon Chicken

Servings: 1
Cooking Time: 15 Minutes
Ingredients:

- 1 chicken breast, boneless and skinless
- 1 fresh lemon juice
- 1 fresh lemon, sliced
- 1/2 tbsp Italian seasoning
- Pepper
- Salt

Directions:

1. Fit the Breville Smart oven with the rack in position
2. Season chicken with Italian season, pepper, and salt.
3. Place chicken breast in baking dish.
4. Pour lemon juice over chicken and arrange lemon slices on top of chicken.
5. Set to bake at 350 F for 20 minutes. After 5 minutes place the baking dish in the preheated oven.
6. Serve and enjoy.

- **Nutrition Info:** Calories 178 Fat 5.4 g Carbohydrates 7.2 g Sugar 3.1 g Protein 24.8 g Cholesterol 77 mg

163. Air Fryer Chicken Tenders

Servings: 4
Cooking Time: 16 Minutes
Ingredients:

- 1 lb chicken tenders
- For rub:
- 1/2 tbsp dried thyme
- 1 tbsp garlic powder
- 1 tbsp paprika
- 1/2 tbsp onion powder
- 1/2 tsp cayenne pepper
- Pepper
- Salt

Directions:

1. Fit the Breville Smart oven with the rack in position 2.
2. In a bowl, add all rub ingredients and mix well.
3. Add chicken tenders into the bowl and coat well.
4. Place chicken tenders in the air fryer basket then place an air fryer basket in the baking pan.
5. Place a baking pan on the oven rack. Set to air fry at 370 F for 16 minutes.
6. Serve and enjoy.
- **Nutrition Info:** Calories 232 Fat 8.7 g Carbohydrates 3.6 g Sugar 1 g Protein 33.6 g Cholesterol 101 mg

164.Super Lemon Chicken

Servings:6
Cooking Time: 35 Minutes
Ingredients:
- 3 (8-ounce / 227-g) boneless, skinless chicken breasts, halved, rinsed
- 1 cup dried bread crumbs
- ¼ cup olive oil
- ¼ cup chicken broth
- Zest of 1 lemon
- 3 medium garlic cloves, minced
- ½ cup fresh lemon juice
- ½ cup water
- ¼ cup minced fresh oregano
- 1 medium lemon, cut into wedges
- ¼ cup minced fresh parsley, divided
- Cooking spray

Directions:
1. Pour the bread crumbs in a shadow dish, then roll the chicken breasts in the bread crumbs to coat.
2. Spritz a skillet with cooking spray, and brown the coated chicken breasts over medium heat about 3 minutes on each side. Transfer the browned chicken to the baking pan.
3. In a small bowl, combine the remaining ingredients, except the lemon and parsley. Pour the sauce over the chicken.
4. Slide the baking pan into Rack Position 1, select Convection Bake, set the temperature

to 325ºF (163ºC) and set the time to 30 minutes.
5. After 15 minutes, remove the pan from the oven. Flip the breasts. Return the pan to the oven and continue cooking.
6. When cooking is complete, the chicken should no longer pink.
7. Transfer to a serving platter, and spoon the sauce over the chicken. Garnish with the lemon and parsley.

165.Deep Fried Duck Leg Quarters

Servings:4
Cooking Time: 45 Minutes
Ingredients:
- 4 (½-pound / 227-g) skin-on duck leg quarters
- 2 medium garlic cloves, minced
- ½ teaspoon salt
- ½ teaspoon ground black pepper

Directions:
1. Spritz the air fryer basket with cooking spray.
2. On a clean work surface, rub the duck leg quarters with garlic, salt, and black pepper.
3. Arrange the leg quarters in the basket and spritz with cooking spray.
4. Put the air fryer basket on the baking pan and slide into Rack Position 2, select Air Fry, set temperature to 300ºF (150ºC) and set time to 30 minutes.
5. After 30 minutes, remove from the oven. Flip the leg quarters. Increase temperature to 375ºF (190ºC) and set time to 15 minutes. Return to the oven and continue cooking.
6. When cooking is complete, the leg quarters should be well browned and crispy.
7. Remove the duck leg quarters from the oven and allow to cool for 10 minutes before serving.

166.Chinese Braised Pork Belly

Servings: 8
Cooking Time: 20 Minutes
Ingredients:
- 1 lb Pork Belly, sliced
- 1 Tbsp Oyster Sauce

- 1 Tbsp Sugar
- 2 Red Fermented Bean Curds
- 1 Tbsp Red Fermented Bean Curd Paste
- 1 Tbsp Cooking Wine
- 1/2 Tbsp Soy Sauce
- 1 Tsp Sesame Oil
- 1 Cup All Purpose Flour

Directions:

1. Preparing the Ingredients. Preheat the Breville Smart air fryer oven to 390 degrees.
2. In a small bowl, mix all ingredients together and rub the pork thoroughly with this mixture
3. Set aside to marinate for at least 30 minutes or preferably overnight for the flavors to permeate the meat
4. Coat each marinated pork belly slice in flour and place in the Breville Smart air fryer oven tray
5. Air Frying. Cook for 15 to 20 minutes until crispy and tender.

167.Cayenne Chicken With Coconut Flakes

Servings: 4
Cooking Time: 25 Minutes
Ingredients:
- 3 chicken breasts, cubed
- 3 cups coconut flakes
- 3 whole eggs, beaten
- ½ cup cornstarch
- Salt and black pepper to taste
- 1 tbsp cayenne pepper

Directions:

1. In a bowl, mix salt, cornstarch, cayenne and black peppers. In another bowl, mix beaten eggs with coconut flakes. Dip the chicken in pepper mix, then in the egg mix. Cover with foil and place in the basket. Fit in the baking tray and cook for 20 minutes at 350 F on Air Fry function.

168.Chicken And Sweet Potato Curry

Servings:4
Cooking Time: 20 Minutes
Ingredients:
- 1 pound (454 g) boneless, skinless chicken thighs
- 1 teaspoon kosher salt, divided

- ¼ cup unsalted butter, melted
- 1 tablespoon curry powder
- 2 medium sweet potatoes, peeled and cut in 1-inch cubes
- 12 ounces (340 g) Brussels sprouts, halved

Directions:

1. Sprinkle the chicken thighs with ½ teaspoon of kosher salt. Place them in the single layer in the baking pan.
2. In a small bowl, stir together the butter and curry powder.
3. Place the sweet potatoes and Brussels sprouts in a large bowl. Drizzle half the curry butter over the vegetables and add the remaining kosher salt. Toss to coat. Transfer the vegetables to the baking pan and place in a single layer around the chicken. Brush half of the remaining curry butter over the chicken.
4. Slide the baking pan into Rack Position 2, select Roast, set temperature to 400ºF (205ºC), and set time to 20 minutes.
5. After 10 minutes, remove from the oven and turn over the chicken thighs. Baste them with the remaining curry butter. Return to the oven and continue cooking.
6. Cooking is complete when the sweet potatoes are tender and the chicken is cooked through and reads 165ºF (74ºC) on a meat thermometer.

169.Roasted Pork Tenderloin

Servings: 4
Cooking Time: 1 Hour
Ingredients:
- 1 (3-pound) pork tenderloin
- 2 tablespoons extra-virgin olive oil
- 2 garlic cloves, minced
- 1 teaspoon dried basil
- 1 teaspoon dried oregano
- 1 teaspoon dried thyme
- Salt
- Pepper

Directions:

1. Preparing the Ingredients. Drizzle the pork tenderloin with the olive oil.

2. Rub the garlic, basil, oregano, thyme, and salt and pepper to taste all over the tenderloin.
3. Air Frying. Place the tenderloin in the Breville Smart air fryer oven. Cook for 45 minutes.
4. Use a meat thermometer to test for doneness
5. Open the Breville Smart air fryer oven and flip the pork tenderloin. Cook for an additional 15 minutes.
6. Remove the cooked pork from the air fryer oven and allow it to rest for 10 minutes before cutting.
- **Nutrition Info:** CALORIES: 283; FAT: 10G; PROTEIN:48

170.Pork Sausage With Cauliflower Mash

Servings:6
Cooking Time: 27 Minutes
Ingredients:
- 1 pound (454 g) cauliflower, chopped
- 6 pork sausages, chopped
- ½ onion, sliced
- 3 eggs, beaten
- $^1/_3$ cup Colby cheese
- 1 teaspoon cumin powder
- ½ teaspoon tarragon
- ½ teaspoon sea salt
- ½ teaspoon ground black pepper
- Cooking spray

Directions:
1. Spritz the baking pan with cooking spray.
2. In a saucepan over medium heat, boil the cauliflower until tender. Place the boiled cauliflower in a food processor and pulse until puréed. Transfer to a large bowl and combine with remaining ingredients until well blended.
3. Pour the cauliflower and sausage mixture into the pan.
4. Slide the baking pan into Rack Position 1, select Convection Bake, set temperature to 365ºF (185ºC) and set time to 27 minutes.
5. When cooking is complete, the sausage should be lightly browned.
6. Divide the mixture among six serving dishes and serve warm.

171.Sweet Asian Chicken Wings

Servings:4
Cooking Time: 25 Minutes
Ingredients:
- 1 lb chicken wings
- 1 cup flour
- 1 cup breadcrumbs
- 2 eggs, beaten
- 2 tbsp canola oil
- Salt and black pepper to taste
- 2 tbsp sesame seeds
- 2 tbsp Korean red pepper paste
- 1 tbsp apple cider vinegar
- 2 tbsp honey
- 1 tbsp soy sauce

Directions:
1. Preheat Breville on AirFry function to 390 F. Separate the chicken wings into winglets and drumettes. In a bowl, mix oil, salt, and pepper. Coat chicken with flour, followed by eggs and breadcrumbs. Place it in the basket. Spray with a bit of oil and press Start. Cook for 15 minutes.
2. Mix red pepper paste, apple cider vinegar, soy sauce, honey, and ¼ cup water in a saucepan over medium heat and bring the mixture to a boil. Add in the chicken and toss to coat. Garnish with sesame seeds and serve.

172.Italian Sausages And Red Grapes

Servings:6
Cooking Time: 20 Minutes
Ingredients:
- 2 pounds (905 g) seedless red grapes
- 3 shallots, sliced
- 2 teaspoons fresh thyme
- 2 tablespoons olive oil
- ½ teaspoon kosher salt
- Freshly ground black pepper, to taste
- 6 links (about 1½ pounds / 680 g) hot Italian sausage
- 3 tablespoons balsamic vinegar

Directions:
1. Place the grapes in a large bowl. Add the shallots, thyme, olive oil, salt, and pepper. Gently toss. Place the grapes in the baking

pan. Arrange the sausage links evenly in the pan.

2. Slide the baking pan into Rack Position 2, select Roast, set temperature to 375ºF (190ºC), and set time to 20 minutes.
3. After 10 minutes, remove the pan. Turn over the sausages and sprinkle the vinegar over the sausages and grapes. Gently toss the grapes and move them to one side of the pan. Return the pan to the oven and continue cooking.
4. When cooking is complete, the grapes should be very soft and the sausages browned. Serve immediately.

173.Ginger Chicken Wings

Servings: 3
Cooking Time: 25 Minutes
Ingredients:
- 1 pound chicken wings
- 1 tbsp cilantro
- Salt and black pepper to taste
- 1 garlic clove, minced
- 1 tbsp yogurt
- 2 tbsp honey
- ½ tbsp vinegar
- ½ tbsp ginger, minced

Directions:
1. Preheat Breville Smart on Air Fry to 360 F. Season wings with salt and pepper, place them in the basket and fit in the baking tray. Cook for 15 minutes, shaking once. In a bowl, mix the remaining ingredients. Top the chicken with sauce and cook for 5 more minutes. Serve.

174.Pork Cutlet Rolls

Servings: 4
Cooking Time: 15 Minutes
Ingredients:
- 4 Pork Cutlets
- 4 Sundried Tomatoes in oil
- 2 Tbsps Parsley, finely chopped
- 1 Green Onion, finely chopped
- Black Pepper to taste
- 2 Tsps Paprika
- 1/2 Tbsp Olive Oil
- * String for Rolled Meat

Directions:
1. Preparing the Ingredients. Preheat the Breville Smart air fryer oven to 390 degrees
2. Finely chop the tomatoes and mix with the parsley and green onion. Add salt and pepper to taste
3. Spread out the cutlets and coat them with the tomato mixture. Roll up the cutlets and secure intact with the string
4. Rub the rolls with salt, pepper, and paprika powder and thinly coat them with olive oil
5. Air Frying. Put the cutlet rolls in the Breville Smart air fryer oven tray and cook for 15 minutes. Roast until nicely brown and done.
6. Serve with tomato sauce.

175.Yakitori

Servings:4
Cooking Time: 15 Minutes
Ingredients:
- ½ cup mirin
- ¼ cup dry white wine
- ½ cup soy sauce
- 1 tablespoon light brown sugar
- 1½ pounds (680 g) boneless, skinless chicken thighs, cut into 1½-inch pieces, fat trimmed
- 4 medium scallions, trimmed, cut into 1½-inch pieces
- Cooking spray

Directions:
1. Special Equipment:
2. (4-inch) bamboo skewers, soaked in water for at least 30 minutes
3. Combine the mirin, dry white wine, soy sauce, and brown sugar in a saucepan. Bring to a boil over medium heat. Keep stirring.
4. Boil for another 2 minutes or until it has a thick consistency. Turn off the heat.
5. Spritz the air fryer basket with cooking spray.
6. Run the bamboo skewers through the chicken pieces and scallions alternatively.
7. Arrange the skewers in the basket, then brush with mirin mixture on both sides. Spritz with cooking spray.
8. Put the air fryer basket on the baking pan and slide into Rack Position 2, select Air Fry,

set temperature to 400ºF (205ºC) and set time to 10 minutes.

9. Flip the skewers halfway through.
10. When cooking is complete, the chicken and scallions should be glossy.
11. Serve immediately.

176.Duck Liver Fries

Servings:x
Cooking Time:x
Ingredients:
- A pinch of salt to taste
- 1 tbsp. lemon juice
- For the garnish:
- 1 cup melted cheddar cheese
- 1 lb. duck liver (Cut in to long Oregano Fingers)
- ingredients for the marinade:
- 1 tbsp. olive oil
- 1 tsp. mixed herbs
- ½ tsp. red chili flakes

Directions:
1. Take all the ingredients mentioned under the heading "For the marinade" and mix them well.
2. Cook the duck liver Oregano Fingers and soak them in the marinade.
3. Pre heat the Breville smart oven for around 5 minutes at 300 Fahrenheit. Take out the basket of the fryer and place the chicken Oregano Fingers in them. Close the basket.
4. Now keep the fryer at 220 Fahrenheit for 20 or 25 minutes. In between the process, toss the fries twice or thrice so that they get cooked properly.
5. Towards the end of the cooking process (the last 2 minutes or so), sprinkle the cut coriander leaves on the fries. Add the melted cheddar cheese over the fries and serve hot.

177.Lime Chicken With Cilantro

Servings:4
Cooking Time: 10 Minutes
Ingredients:
- 4 (4-ounce / 113-g) boneless, skinless chicken breasts
- ½ cup chopped fresh cilantro
- Juice of 1 lime
- Chicken seasoning or rub, to taste
- Salt and ground black pepper, to taste
- Cooking spray

Directions:
1. Put the chicken breasts in the large bowl, then add the cilantro, lime juice, chicken seasoning, salt, and black pepper. Toss to coat well.
2. Wrap the bowl in plastic and refrigerate to marinate for at least 30 minutes.
3. Spritz the air fryer basket with cooking spray.
4. Remove the marinated chicken breasts from the bowl and place in the basket. Spritz with cooking spray.
5. Put the air fryer basket on the baking pan and slide into Rack Position 2, select Air Fry, set temperature to 400ºF (205ºC) and set time to 10 minutes.
6. Flip the breasts halfway through.
7. When cooking is complete, the internal temperature of the chicken should reach at least 165ºF (74ºC).
8. Serve immediately.

178.Mutton Oregano Fingers

Servings:x
Cooking Time:x
Ingredients:
- 1 lb. boneless mutton cut into Oregano Fingers
- 2 tsp. salt
- 1 tsp. pepper powder
- 1 tsp. red chili powder
- 6 tbsp. corn flour
- 2 cup dry breadcrumbs
- 2 tsp. oregano
- 2 tsp. red chili flakes
- 1 ½ tbsp. ginger-garlic paste
- 4 tbsp. lemon juice
- 4 eggs

Directions:
1. Mix all the ingredients for the marinade and put the mutton Oregano Fingers inside and let it rest overnight. Mix the breadcrumbs, oregano and red chili flakes well and place

the marinated Oregano Fingers on this mixture.

2. Cover it with plastic wrap and leave it till right before you serve to cook. Pre heat the Breville smart oven at 160 degrees Fahrenheit for 5 minutes.
3. Place the Oregano Fingers in the fry basket and close it. Let them cook at the same temperature for another 15 minutes or so. Toss the Oregano Fingers well so that they are cooked uniformly.

179.Meatballs(7)

Servings: 4
Cooking Time: 10 Minutes
Ingredients:
- 2 eggs
- 1 tsp sesame oil
- 1 tsp ginger, minced
- 1 tsp garlic, minced
- 1/2 cup breadcrumbs
- 2 lbs ground pork
- 1/3 tsp red chili pepper flakes
- 1 tbsp scallions, diced
- 1 tsp soy sauce
- Pepper
- Salt

Directions:
1. Fit the Breville Smart oven with the rack in position 2.
2. Add all ingredients into the large bowl and mix until well combined.
3. Make small balls from meat mixture and place in the air fryer basket then place the air fryer basket in the baking pan.
4. Place a baking pan on the oven rack. Set to air fry at 400 F for 10 minutes.
5. Serve and enjoy.
- **Nutrition Info:** Calories 423 Fat 12 g Carbohydrates 10.7 g Sugar 1.1 g Protein 64.1 g Cholesterol 247 mg

180.Lamb Chili With Red Chili Sauce

Servings:x
Cooking Time:x
Ingredients:
- 1 lb. lamb (Cut into cubes)
- 2 ½ tsp. ginger-garlic paste

- 1 tsp. red chili sauce
- 2 tbsp. tomato ketchup
- 2 tsp. soya sauce
- 1-2 tbsp. honey
- ¼ tsp. Ajinomoto
- 1-2 tsp. red chili flakes
- ¼ tsp. salt
- ¼ tsp. red chili powder/black pepper
- A few drops of edible orange food coloring
- For sauce:
- 2 tbsp. olive oil
- 1 ½ tsp. ginger garlic paste
- ½ tbsp. red chili sauce

Directions:
1. Mix all the ingredients for the marinade and put the lamb cubes inside and let it rest overnight. Mix the breadcrumbs, oregano and red chili flakes well and place the marinated Oregano Fingers on this mixture. Cover it with plastic wrap and leave it till right before you serve to cook.
2. Pre heat the Breville smart oven at 160 degrees Fahrenheit for 5 minutes. Place the Oregano Fingers in the fry basket and close it. Let them cook at the same temperature for another 15 minutes or so.
3. Toss the Oregano Fingers well so that they are cooked uniformly.

181.Beef And Spinach Meatloaves

Servings:2
Cooking Time: 45 Minutes
Ingredients:
- 1 large egg, beaten
- 1 cup frozen spinach
- $^1/_3$ cup almond meal
- ¼ cup chopped onion
- ¼ cup plain Greek milk
- ¼ teaspoon salt
- ¼ teaspoon dried sage
- 2 teaspoons olive oil, divided
- Freshly ground black pepper, to taste
- ½ pound (227 g) extra-lean ground beef
- ¼ cup tomato paste
- 1 tablespoon granulated stevia
- ¼ teaspoon Worcestershire sauce
- Cooking spray

Directions:

1. Coat a shallow baking pan with cooking spray.
2. In a large bowl, combine the beaten egg, spinach, almond meal, onion, milk, salt, sage, 1 teaspoon of olive oil, and pepper.
3. Crumble the beef over the spinach mixture. Mix well to combine. Divide the meat mixture in half. Shape each half into a loaf. Place the loaves in the prepared pan.
4. In a small bowl, whisk together the tomato paste, stevia, Worcestershire sauce, and remaining 1 teaspoon of olive oil. Spoon half of the sauce over each meatloaf.
5. Slide the baking pan into Rack Position 1, select Convection Bake, set the temperature to 350ºF (180ºC) and set the time to 40 minutes.
6. When cooking is complete, an instant-read thermometer inserted in the center of the meatloaves should read at least 165ºF (74ºC).
7. Serve immediately.

182.Chicken Fried Baked Pastry

Servings:x
Cooking Time:x
Ingredients:

- 1 or 2 green chilies that are finely chopped or mashed
- ½ tsp. cumin
- 1 tsp. coarsely crushed coriander
- 1 dry red chili broken into pieces
- A small amount of salt (to taste)
- 2 tbsp. unsalted butter
- 1 ½ cup all-purpose flour
- A pinch of salt to taste
- Add as much water as required to make the dough stiff and firm
- 1 lb. chicken (Remove the chicken from the bone and cut it into pieces)
- ¼ cup boiled peas
- 1 tsp. powdered ginger
- ½ tsp. dried mango powder
- ½ tsp. red chili power.
- 1-2 tbsp. coriander.

Directions:

1. You will first need to make the outer covering. In a large bowl, add the flour, butter and enough water to knead it into dough that is stiff. Transfer this to a container and leave it to rest for five minutes.
2. Place a pan on medium flame and add the oil. Roast the mustard seeds and once roasted, add the coriander seeds and the chopped dry red chilies. Add all the dry ingredients for the filling and mix the ingredients well.
3. Add a little water and continue to stir the ingredients. Make small balls out of the dough and roll them out. Cut the rolled-out dough into halves and apply a little water on the edges to help you fold the halves into a cone. Add the filling to the cone and close up the samosa. Pre-heat the Breville smart oven for around 5 to 6 minutes at 300 Fahrenheit.
4. Place all the samosas in the fry basket and close the basket properly. Keep the Breville smart oven at 200 degrees for another 20 to 25 minutes. Around the halfway point, open the basket and turn the samosas over for uniform cooking.
5. After this, fry at 250 degrees for around 10 minutes in order to give them the desired golden-brown color. Serve hot. Recommended sides are tamarind or mint sauce.

183.Juicy Baked Chicken Breast

Servings: 4
Cooking Time: 25 Minutes
Ingredients:

- 4 chicken breasts
- 1 tbsp fresh parsley, chopped
- 1/4 tsp red pepper flakes
- 1/2 tsp black pepper
- 1 tsp Italian seasoning
- 2 tbsp olive oil
- 1/4 cup balsamic vinegar
- 1 tsp kosher salt

Directions:

1. Fit the Breville Smart oven with the rack in position

2. Place chicken breasts into the mixing bowl.
3. Mix together remaining ingredients and pour over chicken breasts and coat well and let marinate for 30 minutes.
4. Arrange marinated chicken breasts into a greased baking dish.
5. Set to bake at 425 F for 30 minutes. After 5 minutes place the baking dish in the preheated oven.
6. Slice and serve.
- **Nutrition Info:** Calories 345 Fat 18.2 g Carbohydrates 0.6 g Sugar 0.2 g Protein 42.3 g Cholesterol 131 mg

184.Veal Club Classic Sandwich

Servings:x
Cooking Time:x
Ingredients:
- 2 slices of white bread
- 1 tbsp. softened butter
- ½ tsp. olive oil
- ½ flake garlic crushed
- ¼ cup chopped onion
- ¼ tsp. mustard powder
- ½ tbsp. sugar
- ¼ tbsp. red chili sauce
- ½ lb. cubed veal
- 1 small capsicum
- ¼ tbsp. Worcestershire sauce
- ½ cup water

Directions:
1. Take the slices of bread and remove the edges. Now cut the slices horizontally. Cook the ingredients for the sauce and wait till it thickens. Now, add the veal to the sauce and stir till it obtains the flavors. Roast the capsicum and peel the skin off. Cut the capsicum into slices. Mix the ingredients together and apply it to the bread slices.
2. Pre-heat the Breville smart oven for 5 minutes at 300 Fahrenheit. Open the basket of the Fryer and place the prepared Classic Sandwiches in it such that no two Classic Sandwiches are touching each other. Now keep the fryer at 250 degrees for around 15 minutes. Turn the Classic Sandwiches in between the cooking process to cook both

slices. Serve the Classic Sandwiches with tomato ketchup or mint sauce.

185.Baked Beef & Broccoli

Servings: 2
Cooking Time: 25 Minutes
Ingredients:
- 1/2 lb beef meat, cut into pieces
- 1 tbsp vinegar
- 1 garlic clove, minced
- 1 tbsp olive oil
- 1/2 tsp Italian seasoning
- 1/2 cup broccoli florets
- 1 onion, sliced
- Pepper
- Salt

Directions:
1. Fit the Breville Smart oven with the rack in position
2. Add meat and remaining ingredients into the large bowl and toss well and spread in baking pan.
3. Set to bake at 390 F for 30 minutes. After 5 minutes place the baking pan in the preheated oven.
4. Serve and enjoy.
- **Nutrition Info:** Calories 316 Fat 16.1 g Carbohydrates 7.4 g Sugar 2.9 g Protein 34.4 g Cholesterol 102 mg

186.Amazing Bacon & Potato Platter

Servings: 4
Cooking Time: 40 Minutes
Ingredients:
- 4 potatoes, halved
- 6 garlic cloves, squashed
- 4 streaky cut rashers bacon
- 1 tbsp olive oil

Directions:
1. In a mixing bowl, mix garlic, bacon, potatoes, and olive oil; toss to coat. Place the mixture in the basket and fit in the baking tray; roast for 25-30 minutes at 400 F on Air Fry, shaking once.

187.Sherry Grilled Chicken

Servings: 2
Cooking Time: 25 Minutes

Ingredients:
- 2 chicken breasts, cubed
- 2 garlic clove, minced
- ½ cup ketchup
- ½ tbsp ginger, minced
- ½ cup soy sauce
- 2 tbsp sherry
- ½ cup pineapple juice
- 2 tbsp apple cider vinegar
- ½ cup brown sugar

Directions:
1. In a bowl, mix ketchup, pineapple juice, sugar, cider vinegar, and ginger. Heat the mixture in a frying pan over low heat. Cover chicken with the soy sauce and sherry; pour the hot sauce on top. Set aside for 15 minutes to marinate.
2. Preheat your Breville Smart oven on Broil function to 360 F. Remove the chicken from the marinade, pat dry, and place it in the greased basket. Fit in a baking tray and cook for 15 minutes.

188.Baked Pork Ribs

Servings: 8
Cooking Time: 30 Minutes
Ingredients:
- 2 lbs pork ribs, boneless
- 1 tbsp onion powder
- 1 1/2 tbsp garlic powder
- Pepper
- Salt

Directions:
1. Fit the Breville Smart oven with the rack in position
2. Place pork ribs in baking pan and season with onion powder, garlic powder, pepper, and salt.
3. Set to bake at 350 F for 35 minutes. After 5 minutes place the baking pan in the preheated oven.
4. Serve and enjoy.
- **Nutrition Info:** Calories 318 Fat 20.1 g Carbohydrates 1.9 g Sugar 0.7 g Protein 30.4 g Cholesterol 117 mg

189.Bacon-wrapped Turkey With Carrots

Servings:4

Cooking Time: 25 Minutes
Ingredients:
- 2 (12-ounce / 340-g) turkey tenderloins
- 1 teaspoon kosher salt, divided
- 6 slices bacon
- 3 tablespoons balsamic vinegar
- 2 tablespoons honey
- 1 tablespoon Dijon mustard
- ½ teaspoon dried thyme
- 6 large carrots, peeled and cut into ¼-inch rounds
- 1 tablespoon olive oil

Directions:
1. Sprinkle the turkey with ¾ teaspoon of the salt. Wrap each tenderloin with 3 strips of bacon, securing the bacon with toothpicks. Place the turkey in the baking pan.
2. In a small bowl, mix the balsamic vinegar, honey, mustard, and thyme.
3. Place the carrots in a medium bowl and drizzle with the oil. Add 1 tablespoon of the balsamic mixture and ¼ teaspoon of kosher salt and toss to coat. Place these on the pan around the turkey tenderloins. Baste the tenderloins with about one-half of the remaining balsamic mixture.
4. Slide the baking pan into Rack Position 2, select Roast, set temperature to 375ºF (190ºC), and set time to 25 minutes.
5. After 13 minutes, remove from the oven. Gently stir the carrots. Flip the tenderloins and baste with the remaining balsamic mixture. Return the pan to the oven and continue cooking.
6. When cooking is complete, the carrots should tender and the center of the tenderloins should register 165ºF (74ºC) on a meat thermometer. Remove from the oven. Slice the turkey and serve with the carrots.

190.Mango Marinated Chicken Breasts

Servings: 2
Cooking Time: 20 Minutes + Marinating Time
Ingredients:
- 2 chicken breasts, cubed
- 1 large mango, cubed
- 1 red pepper, chopped
- 2 tbsp balsamic vinegar

- 5 tbsp olive oil
- 2 garlic cloves, minced
- 1 tbsp fresh parsley, chopped
- Salt to taste

Directions:
1. In a bowl, mix mango, garlic, red pepper, olive oil, salt, and balsamic vinegar. Add the mixture to a blender and pulse until smooth. Transfer to a bowl and add in the chicken cubes. Toss to coat and place in the fridge for 30 minutes.
2. Preheat Breville Smart on Air Fry function to 360 F. Remove the chicken from the fridge and place cubes in the greased basket. Fit in the baking tray and cook in the air fryer oven for 12 minutes, shaking once. Garnish with parsley and serve.

191.Cheesy Chicken Tenders

Servings: 4
Cooking Time: 30 Minutes
Ingredients:
- 1 large white meat chicken breast, approximately 5-6 ounces, sliced into strips
- 1 cup of breadcrumbs (Panko brand works well)
- 2 medium-sized eggs
- Pinch of salt and pepper
- 1 tablespoon of grated or powdered parmesan cheese

Directions:
1. Preparing the Ingredients. Cover the basket of the Breville Smart air fryer oven with a lining of tin foil, leaving the edges uncovered to allow air to circulate through the basket. Preheat the Breville Smart air fryer oven to 350 degrees. In a mixing bowl, beat the eggs until fluffy and until the yolks and whites are fully combined, and set aside. In a separate mixing bowl, combine the breadcrumbs, parmesan, salt, and pepper, and set aside. One by one, dip each piece of raw chicken into the bowl with dry ingredients, coating all sides; then submerge into the bowl with wet ingredients, then dip again into the dry ingredients. Lay the coated chicken pieces on the foil covering the Oven rack/basket,

in a single flat layer. Place the Rack on the middle-shelf of the Breville Smart air fryer oven.
2. Air Frying. Set the Breville Smart air fryer oven timer for 15 minutes. After 15 minutes, the air fryer will turn off and the chicken should be mid-way cooked and the breaded coating starting to brown. Using tongs turn each piece of chicken over to ensure a full all over fry. Reset the air fryer oven to 320 degrees for another 15 minutes. After 15 minutes, when the air fryer shuts off, remove the fried chicken strips using tongs and set on a serving plate. Eat as soon as cool enough to handle, and enjoy!
- **Nutrition Info:** CALORIES: 278; FAT: 15G; PROTEIN:29G; SUGAR:7G

192.Easy Pork Chops With Italian Herbs

Servings:4
Cooking Time: 30 Minutes
Ingredients:
- 4 pork chops
- 2 tbsp olive oil
- Salt and black pepper to taste
- 2 eggs, beaten
- 1 tbsp flour
- Breadcrumbs as needed
- 1 tsp dried Italian herbs

Directions:
1. in a bowl, mix olive oil, salt, and pepper. Place the beaten egg in a plate. In a separate plate, add the breadcrumbs. Coat the pork with the oil and allow to rest for 15 minutes.
2. Dip the chops in the eggs and roll in the breadcrumbs. Place the in the cooking basket. Select AirFry function, adjust the temperature to 390 F, and press Start. Cook for 20 minutes.

193.Mayo Chicken Breasts With Basil & Cheese

Servings:4
Cooking Time: 20 Minutes
Ingredients:
- 4 chicken breasts, cubed
- 1 tsp garlic powder

- 1 cup mayonnaise
- Salt and black pepper to taste
- ½ cup cream cheese, softened
- Chopped basil for garnish

Directions:
1. In a bowl, mix cream cheese, mayonnaise, garlic powder, and salt. Add in the chicken and toss to coat. Place the chicken in the basket and Press Start. Cook for 15 minutes at 380 F on AirFry function. Serve garnished with roughly chopped fresh basil.

194.Golden Chicken Cutlets

Servings:4
Cooking Time: 15 Minutes
Ingredients:
- 2 tablespoons panko bread crumbs
- ¼ cup grated Parmesan cheese
- ⅛ tablespoon paprika
- ½ tablespoon garlic powder
- 2 large eggs
- 4 chicken cutlets
- 1 tablespoon parsley
- Salt and ground black pepper, to taste
- Cooking spray

Directions:
1. Spritz the air fryer basket with cooking spray.
2. Combine the bread crumbs, Parmesan, paprika, garlic powder, salt, and ground black pepper in a large bowl. Stir to mix well. Beat the eggs in a separate bowl.
3. Dredge the chicken cutlets in the beaten eggs, then roll over the bread crumbs mixture to coat well. Shake the excess off.
4. Transfer the chicken cutlets in the basket and spritz with cooking spray.
5. Put the air fryer basket on the baking pan and slide into Rack Position 2, select Air Fry, set temperature to 400ºF (205ºC) and set time to 15 minutes.
6. Flip the cutlets halfway through.
7. When cooking is complete, the cutlets should be crispy and golden brown.
8. Serve with parsley on top.

195.Flavors Cheesy Chicken Breasts

Servings: 6
Cooking Time: 45 Minutes
Ingredients:
- 3 lbs chicken breasts, sliced in half
- 1 tsp garlic powder
- 1/2 cup parmesan cheese, shredded
- 1 cup Greek yogurt
- 1/2 tsp pepper
- 1/2 tsp salt

Directions:
1. Fit the Breville Smart oven with the rack in position
2. Place chicken breasts into the greased baking dish.
3. Mix parmesan cheese, yogurt, garlic powder, pepper, and salt and pour over chicken.
4. Set to bake at 375 F for 50 minutes. After 5 minutes place the baking dish in the preheated oven.
5. Serve and enjoy.
- **Nutrition Info:** Calories 482 Fat 19.1 g Carbohydrates 2.1 g Sugar 1.5 g Protein 71.5 g Cholesterol 209 mg

FISH & SEAFOOD RECIPES

196.Roasted Scallops With Snow Peas

Servings:4
Cooking Time: 8 Minutes
Ingredients:

- 1 pound (454 g) sea scallops
- 3 tablespoons hoisin sauce
- ½ cup toasted sesame seeds
- 6 ounces (170 g) snow peas, trimmed
- 3 teaspoons vegetable oil, divided
- 1 teaspoon soy sauce
- 1 teaspoon sesame oil
- 1 cup roasted mushrooms

Directions:

1. Brush the scallops with the hoisin sauce. Put the sesame seeds in a shallow dish. Roll the scallops in the sesame seeds until evenly coated.
2. Combine the snow peas with 1 teaspoon of vegetable oil, the sesame oil, and soy sauce in a medium bowl and toss to coat.
3. Grease the baking pan with the remaining 2 teaspoons of vegetable oil. Put the scallops in the middle of the pan and arrange the snow peas around the scallops in a single layer.
4. Slide the baking pan into Rack Position 2, select Roast, set temperature to 375ºF (190ºC), and set time to 8 minutes.
5. After 5 minutes, remove the pan and flip the scallops. Fold in the mushrooms and stir well. Return the pan to the oven and continue cooking.
6. When done, remove from the oven and cool for 5 minutes. Serve warm.

197.Tropical Shrimp Skewers

Servings: 4
Cooking Time: 5 Minutes
Ingredients:

- 1 tbsp. lime juice
- 1 tbsp. honey
- ¼ tsp red pepper flakes
- ¼ tsp pepper
- ¼ tsp ginger
- Nonstick cooking spray
- 1 lb. medium shrimp, peel, devein & leave tails on
- 2 cups peaches, drain & chop
- ½ green bell pepper, chopped fine
- ¼ cup scallions, chopped

Directions:

1. Soak 8 small wooden skewers in water for 15 minutes.
2. In a small bowl, whisk together lime juice, honey and spices. Transfer 2 tablespoons of the mixture to a medium bowl.
3. Place the baking pan in position 2 of the oven. Lightly spray fryer basket with cooking spray. Set oven to broil on 400°F for 10 minutes.
4. Thread 5 shrimp on each skewer and brush both sides with marinade. Place in basket and after 5 minutes, place on the baking pan. Cook 4-5 minutes or until shrimp turn pink.
5. Add peaches, bell pepper, and scallions to reserved honey mixture, mix well. Divide salsa evenly between serving plates and top with 2 skewers each. Serve immediately.
- **Nutrition Info:** Calories 181, Total Fat 1g, Saturated Fat 0g, Total Carbs 27g, Net Carbs 25g, Protein 16g, Sugar 21g, Fiber 2g, Sodium 650mg, Potassium 288mg, Phosphorus 297mg

198.Salmon & Caper Cakes

Servings:2
Cooking Time: 15 Minutes + Chilling Time
Ingredients:

- 8 oz salmon, cooked
- 1 ½ oz potatoes, mashed
- A handful of capers
- 1 tbsp fresh parsley, chopped
- Zest of 1 lemon
- 1 ¾ oz plain flour

Directions:

1. Carefully flake the salmon. In a bowl, mix the salmon, zest, capers, dill, and mashed potatoes. Form small cakes from the mixture and dust them with flour; refrigerate for 60 minutes. Preheat Breville to 350 F. Press Start and cook the cakes for 10 minutes on AirFry function. Serve chilled.

199.Cheesy Tilapia Fillets

Servings: 4

Cooking Time: 15 Minutes

Ingredients:

- ¾ cup grated Parmesan cheese
- 1 tbsp olive oil
- 2 tsp paprika
- 1 tbsp chopped parsley
- ¼ tsp garlic powder
- 4 tilapia fillets

Directions:

1. Preheat Breville Smart on Air Fry function to 350 F. Mix parsley, Parmesan cheese, garlic, and paprika in a bowl. Brush the olive oil over the fillets and then coat with the Parmesan mixture. Place the tilapia onto a lined baking sheet and cook for 8-10 minutes, turning once. Serve.

200.Air Fryer Salmon

Servings: 2

Cooking Time: 10 Minutes

Ingredients:

- ½ tsp. salt
- ½ tsp. garlic powder
- ½ tsp. smoked paprika
- Salmon

Directions:

1. Preparing the Ingredients. Mix spices and sprinkle onto salmon.
2. Place seasoned salmon into the Breville Smart air fryer oven.
3. Air Frying. Set temperature to 400°F, and set time to 10 minutes.
- **Nutrition Info:** CALORIES: 185; FAT: 11G; PROTEIN:21G; SUGAR:0G

201.Orange Fish Fillets

Servings: 2

Cooking Time: 25 Minutes

Ingredients:

- 1 lb salmon fillets
- 1 orange juice
- 1 orange zest, grated
- 2 tbsp honey
- 3 tbsp soy sauce

Directions:

1. Fit the Breville Smart oven with the rack in position
2. In a small bowl, whisk together honey, soy sauce, orange juice, and orange zest.
3. Place salmon fillets in a baking dish and pour honey mixture over salmon fillets.
4. Set to bake at 425 F for 30 minutes. After 5 minutes place the baking dish in the preheated oven.
5. Serve and enjoy.
- **Nutrition Info:** Calories 399 Fat 14.1 g Carbohydrates 24.4 g Sugar 21.3 g Protein 45.9 g Cholesterol 100 mg

202.Sweet Cajun Salmon

Servings: 1

Cooking Time: 10 Minutes

Ingredients:

- 1 salmon fillet
- ¼ tsp brown sugar
- Juice of ½ lemon
- 1 tbsp cajun seasoning
- 2 lemon wedges
- 1 tbsp chopped parsley

Directions:

1. Preheat Breville Smart on Bake function to 350 F. Combine sugar and lemon juice; coat the salmon with this mixture. Coat with the Cajun seasoning as well. Place a parchment paper on a baking tray and cook the fish in your Breville Smart for 10 minutes. Serve with lemon wedges and parsley.

203.Flavorful Herb Salmon

Servings: 4

Cooking Time: 15 Minutes

Ingredients:

- 1 lb salmon fillets
- 1/2 tbsp dried rosemary
- 1 tbsp olive oil
- 1/4 tsp dried basil
- 1 tbsp dried chives
- 1/4 tsp dried thyme
- Pepper
- Salt

Directions:

1. Fit the Breville Smart oven with the rack in position 2.

2. Place salmon skin side down in air fryer basket then place an air fryer basket in baking pan.
3. Mix olive oil, thyme, basil, chives, and rosemary in a small bowl.
4. Brush salmon with oil mixture.
5. Place a baking pan on the oven rack. Set to air fry at 400 F for 15 minutes.
6. Serve and enjoy.
- **Nutrition Info:** Calories 182 Fat 10.6 g Carbohydrates 0.4 g Sugar 0 g Protein 22.1 g Cholesterol 50 mg

204.Coconut Shrimp

Servings: 4
Cooking Time: 5 Minutes
Ingredients:
- 1 (8-ounce) can crushed pineapple
- ½ cup sour cream
- ¼ cup pineapple preserves
- 2 egg whites
- ⅔ cup cornstarch
- ⅔ cup sweetened coconut
- 1 cup panko bread crumbs
- 1 pound uncooked large shrimp, thawed if frozen, deveined and shelled
- Olive oil for misting

Directions:
1. Preparing the Ingredients. Drain the crushed pineapple well, reserving the juice. In a small bowl, combine the pineapple, sour cream, and preserves, and mix well. Set aside. In a shallow bowl, beat the egg whites with 2 tablespoons of the reserved pineapple liquid. Place the cornstarch on a plate. Combine the coconut and bread crumbs on another plate. Dip the shrimp into the cornstarch, shake it off, then dip into the egg white mixture and finally into the coconut mixture. Place the shrimp in the air fryer rack/basket and mist with oil.
2. Air Frying. Air-fry for 5 to 7 minutes or until the shrimp are crisp and golden brown.
- **Nutrition Info:** CALORIES: 524; FAT: 14G; PROTEIN:33G; FIBER:4G

205.Rosemary & Garlic Prawns

Servings:2

Cooking Time: 15 Minutes + Chilling Time
Ingredients:
- 8 large prawns
- 2 garlic cloves, minced
- 1 rosemary sprig, chopped
- 1 tbsp butter, melted
- Salt and black pepper to taste

Directions:
1. Combine garlic, butter, rosemary, salt, and pepper in a bowl. Add in the prawns and mix to coat. Cover the bowl and refrigerate for 1 hour. Preheat Breville on AirFry function to 350 F. Remove the prawns from the fridge and transfer to the frying basket. Cook for 6-8 minutes.

206.Tasty Tuna Loaf

Servings: 6
Cooking Time: 40 Minutes
Ingredients:
- Nonstick cooking spray
- 12 oz. can chunk white tuna in water, drain & flake
- ¾ cup bread crumbs
- 1 onion, chopped fine
- 2 eggs, beaten
- ¼ cup milk
- ½ tsp fresh lemon juice
- ½ tsp dill
- 1 tbsp. fresh parsley, chopped
- ½ tsp salt
- ½ tsp pepper

Directions:
1. Place rack in position 1 of the oven. Spray a 9-inch loaf pan with cooking spray.
2. In a large bowl, combine all ingredients until thoroughly mixed. Spread evenly in prepared pan.
3. Set oven to bake on 350°F for 45 minutes. After 5 minutes, place the pan in the oven and cook 40 minutes, or until top is golden brown. Slice and serve.
- **Nutrition Info:** Calories 169, Total Fat 5g, Saturated Fat 1g, Total Carbs 13g, Net Carbs 12g, Protein 18g, Sugar 3g, Fiber 1g, Sodium 540mg, Potassium 247mg, Phosphorus 202mg

207.Mustard-crusted Sole Fillets

Servings:4
Cooking Time: 10 Minutes
Ingredients:

- 5 teaspoons low-sodium yellow mustard
- 1 tablespoon freshly squeezed lemon juice
- 4 (3.5-ounce / 99-g) sole fillets
- 2 teaspoons olive oil
- ½ teaspoon dried marjoram
- ½ teaspoon dried thyme
- ⅛ teaspoon freshly ground black pepper
- 1 slice low-sodium whole-wheat bread, crumbled

Directions:

1. Whisk together the mustard and lemon juice in a small bowl until thoroughly mixed and smooth. Spread the mixture evenly over the sole fillets, then transfer the fillets to the baking pan.
2. In a separate bowl, combine the olive oil, marjoram, thyme, black pepper, and bread crumbs and stir to mix well. Gently but firmly press the mixture onto the top of fillets, coating them completely.
3. Slide the baking pan into Rack Position 1, select Convection Bake, set temperature to 320ºF (160ºC), and set time to 10 minutes.
4. When cooking is complete, the fish should reach an internal temperature of 145ºF (63ºC) on a meat thermometer. Remove from the oven and serve on a plate.

208.Delicious Shrimp Casserole

Servings: 10
Cooking Time: 30 Minutes
Ingredients:

- 1 lb shrimp, peeled & tail off
- 2 tsp onion powder
- 2 tsp old bay seasoning
- 2 cups cheddar cheese, shredded
- 10.5 oz can cream of mushroom soup
- 12 oz long-grain rice
- 1 tsp salt

Directions:

1. Fit the Breville Smart oven with the rack in position

2. Cook rice according to the packet instructions.
3. Add shrimp into the boiling water and cook for 4 minutes or until cooked. Drain shrimp.
4. In a bowl, mix rice, shrimp, and remaining ingredients and pour into the greased 13*9-inch casserole dish.
5. Set to bake at 350 F for 35 minutes. After 5 minutes place the casserole dish in the preheated oven.
6. Serve and enjoy.
- **Nutrition Info:** Calories 286 Fat 9 g Carbohydrates 31 g Sugar 1 g Protein 18.8 g Cholesterol 120 mg

209.Seafood Pizza

Servings:x
Cooking Time:x
Ingredients:

- One pizza base
- Grated pizza cheese (mozzarella cheese preferably) for topping
- Some pizza topping sauce
- Use cooking oil for brushing and topping purposes
- ingredients for topping:
- 2 onions chopped
- 2 cups mixed seafood
- 2 capsicums chopped
- 2 tomatoes that have been deseeded and chopped
- 1 tbsp. (optional) mushrooms/corns
- 2 tsp. pizza seasoning
- Some cottage cheese that has been cut into small cubes (optional)

Directions:

1. Put the pizza base in a pre-heated Breville smart oven for around 5 minutes. (Pre heated to 340 Fahrenheit). Take out the base. Pour some pizza sauce on top of the base at the center. Using a spoon spread the sauce over the base making sure that you leave some gap around the circumference. Grate some mozzarella cheese and sprinkle it over the sauce layer. Take all the vegetables and the seafood and mix them in a bowl. Add some oil and seasoning.

2. Also add some salt and pepper according to taste. Mix them properly. Put this topping over the layer of cheese on the pizza. Now sprinkle some more grated cheese and pizza seasoning on top of this layer. Pre heat the Breville smart oven at 250 Fahrenheit for around 5 minutes.

3. Open the fry basket and place the pizza inside. Close the basket and keep the fryer at 170 degrees for another 10 minutes. If you feel that it is undercooked you may put it at the same temperature for another 2 minutes or so.

210. Air-fried Scallops

Servings:2
Cooking Time: 12 Minutes
Ingredients:
- $1/_3$ cup shallots, chopped
- 1½ tablespoons olive oil
- 1½ tablespoons coconut aminos
- 1 tablespoon Mediterranean seasoning mix
- ½ tablespoon balsamic vinegar
- ½ teaspoon ginger, grated
- 1 clove garlic, chopped
- 1 pound (454 g) scallops, cleanedCooking spray
- Belgian endive, for garnish

Directions:
1. Place all the ingredients except the scallops and Belgian endive in a small skillet over medium heat and stir to combine. Let this mixture simmer for about 2 minutes.
2. Remove the mixture from the skillet to a large bowl and set aside to cool.
3. Add the scallops, coating them all over, then transfer to the refrigerator to marinate for at least 2 hours.
4. When ready, place the scallops in the air fryer basket in a single layer and spray with cooking spray.
5. Put the air fryer basket on the baking pan and slide into Rack Position 2, select Air Fry, set temperature to 345ºF (174ºC), and set time to 10 minutes.
6. Flip the scallops halfway through the cooking time.

7. When cooking is complete, the scallops should be tender and opaque. Remove from the oven and serve garnished with the Belgian endive.

211. Moist & Juicy Baked Cod

Servings: 2
Cooking Time: 10 Minutes
Ingredients:
- 1 lb cod fillets
- 1 1/2 tbsp olive oil
- 3 dashes cayenne pepper
- 1 tbsp fresh lemon juice
- 1/4 tsp salt

Directions:
1. Fit the Breville Smart oven with the rack in position
2. Place fish fillets in a baking pan.
3. Drizzle with oil and lemon juice and sprinkle with cayenne pepper and salt.
4. Set to bake at 400 F for 15 minutes. After 5 minutes place the baking pan in the preheated oven.
5. Serve and enjoy.
- **Nutrition Info:** Calories 275 Fat 12.7 g Carbohydrates 0.4 g Sugar 0.2 g Protein 40.6 g Cholesterol 111 mg

212. Herb Fish Fillets

Servings: 2
Cooking Time: 5 Minutes
Ingredients:
- 2 salmon fillets
- 1/4 tsp smoked paprika
- 1 tsp herb de Provence
- 1 tbsp butter, melted
- 2 tbsp olive oil
- Pepper
- Salt

Directions:
1. Fit the Breville Smart oven with the rack in position 2.
2. Brush salmon fillets with oil and sprinkle with paprika, herb de Provence, pepper, and salt.
3. Place salmon fillets in the air fryer basket then place an air fryer basket in the baking pan.

4. Place a baking pan on the oven rack. Set to air fry at 390 F for 5 minutes.
5. Drizzle melted butter over salmon and serve.
- **Nutrition Info:** Calories 413 Fat 31.1 g Carbohydrates 0.2 g Sugar 0 g Protein 35.4 g Cholesterol 94 mg

213.Crispy Coated Scallops

Servings: 4
Cooking Time: 10 Minutes
Ingredients:
- Nonstick cooking spray
- 1 lb. sea scallops, patted dry
- 1 teaspoon onion powder
- ½ tsp pepper
- 1 egg
- 1 tbsp. water
- ¼ cup Italian bread crumbs
- Paprika
- 1 tbsp. fresh lemon juice

Directions:
1. Lightly spray fryer basket with cooking spray. Place baking pan in position 2 of the oven.
2. Sprinkle scallops with onion powder and pepper.
3. In a shallow dish, whisk together egg and water.
4. Place bread crumbs in a separate shallow dish.
5. Dip scallops in egg then bread crumbs coating them lightly. Place in fryer basket and lightly spray with cooking spray. Sprinkle with paprika.
6. Place the basket on the baking pan and set oven to air fryer on 400°F. Bake 10-12 minutes until scallops are firm on the inside and golden brown on the outside. Drizzle with lemon juice and serve.
- **Nutrition Info:** Calories 122, Total Fat 2g, Saturated Fat 1g, Total Carbs 10g, Net Carbs 9g, Protein 16g, Sugar 1g, Fiber 1g, Sodium 563mg, Potassium 282mg, Phosphorus 420mg

214.Mediterranean Sole

Servings: 6

Cooking Time: 20 Minutes
Ingredients:
- Nonstick cooking spray
- 2 tbsp. olive oil
- 8 scallions, sliced thin
- 2 cloves garlic, diced fine
- 4 tomatoes, chopped
- ½ cup dry white wine
- 2 tbsp. fresh parsley, chopped fine
- 1 tsp oregano
- 1 tsp pepper
- 2 lbs. sole, cut in 6 pieces
- 4 oz. feta cheese, crumbled

Directions:
1. Place the rack in position 1 of the oven. Spray an 8x11-inch baking dish with cooking spray.
2. Heat the oil in a medium skillet over medium heat. Add scallions and garlic and cook until tender, stirring frequently.
3. Add the tomatoes, wine, parsley, oregano, and pepper. Stir to mix. Simmer for 5 minutes, or until sauce thickens. Remove from heat.
4. Pour half the sauce on the bottom of the prepared dish. Lay fish on top then pour remaining sauce over the top. Sprinkle with feta.
5. Set the oven to bake on 400°F for 25 minutes. After 5 minutes, place the baking dish on the rack and cook 15-18 minutes or until fish flakes easily with a fork. Serve immediately.
- **Nutrition Info:** Calories 220, Total Fat 12g, Saturated Fat 4g, Total Carbs 6g, Net Carbs 4g, Protein 22g, Sugar 4g, Fiber 2g, Sodium 631mg, Potassium 540mg, Phosphorus 478mg

215.Asian-inspired Swordfish Steaks

Servings:4
Cooking Time: 8 Minutes
Ingredients:
- 4 (4-ounce / 113-g) swordfish steaks
- ½ teaspoon toasted sesame oil
- 1 jalapeño pepper, finely minced
- 2 garlic cloves, grated
- 2 tablespoons freshly squeezed lemon juice

- 1 tablespoon grated fresh ginger
- ½ teaspoon Chinese five-spice powder
- ⅛ teaspoon freshly ground black pepper

Directions:
1. On a clean work surface, place the swordfish steaks and brush both sides of the fish with the sesame oil.
2. Combine the jalapeño, garlic, lemon juice, ginger, five-spice powder, and black pepper in a small bowl and stir to mix well. Rub the mixture all over the fish until completely coated. Allow to sit for 10 minutes.
3. When ready, arrange the swordfish steaks in the air fryer basket.
4. Put the air fryer basket on the baking pan and slide into Rack Position 2, select Air Fry, set temperature to 380ºF (193ºC), and set time to 8 minutes.
5. Flip the steaks halfway through.
6. When cooking is complete, remove from the oven and cool for 5 minutes before serving.

216.Flavorful Baked Halibut

Servings: 4
Cooking Time: 12 Minutes
Ingredients:
- 1 lb halibut fillets
- 1/4 tsp garlic powder
- 1/4 tsp paprika
- 1/4 tsp smoked paprika
- 1/4 tsp pepper
- 1/4 cup olive oil
- 1 lemon juice
- 1/2 tsp salt

Directions:
1. Fit the Breville Smart oven with the rack in position
2. Place fish fillets into the baking dish.
3. In a small bowl, mix lemon juice, oil, paprika, smoked paprika, garlic powder, and salt.
4. Brush lemon juice mixture over fish fillets.
5. Set to bake at 425 F for 17 minutes. After 5 minutes place the baking dish in the preheated oven.
6. Serve and enjoy.
- **Nutrition Info:** Calories 236 Fat 15.3 g Carbohydrates 0.4 g Sugar 0.1 g Protein 24 g Cholesterol 36 mg

217.Sesame Seeds Coated Fish

Servings:5
Cooking Time: 8 Minutes
Ingredients:
- 3 tablespoons plain flour
- 2 eggs
- ½ cup sesame seeds, toasted
- ½ cup breadcrumbs
- 1/8 teaspoon dried rosemary, crushed
- Pinch of salt
- Pinch of black pepper
- 3 tablespoons olive oil
- 5 frozen fish fillets (white fish of your choice)

Directions:
1. Preparing the Ingredients. In a shallow dish, place flour. In a second shallow dish, beat the eggs. In a third shallow dish, add remaining ingredients except fish fillets and mix till a crumbly mixture forms.
2. Coat the fillets with flour and shake off the excess flour.
3. Next, dip the fillets in the egg.
4. Then coat the fillets with sesame seeds mixture generously.
5. Preheat the Breville Smart air fryer oven to 390 degrees F.
6. Air Frying. Line an Air fryer rack/basket with a piece of foil. Arrange the fillets into prepared basket.
7. Cook for about 14 minutes, flipping once after 10 minutes.

218.Blackened Tuna Steaks

Servings:x
Cooking Time:x
Ingredients:
- 2 Tbsp canola oil
- 4 (8-oz) tuna steaks, preferably sushi-grade
- Blackening Spice:
- ½ cup freshly ground black pepper
- 2 Tbsp kosher salt
- 1 Tbsp cardamom
- 1 Tbsp ground cinnamon
- 1 Tbsp nutmeg
- 1 Tbsp ground cloves
- 1 tsp coriander

- 1 tsp cumin
- 1 tsp cayenne pepper
- ½ tsp celery salt

Directions:
1. First prepare the blackening spice by combining all the spices.
2. Preheat Breville smart oven.
3. Place oil inside the pot and wait until smoking.
4. Sprinkle blackening mixture on top of both sides of tuna steaks (about
5. -2 Tbsp of blackening spice, depending on how spicy you want your steaks).
6. Add tuna into Breville smart oven and cook about 3 minutes each side. The tuna should be browned on the outside and rare on the inside.

219.Paprika Shrimp

Servings:4
Cooking Time: 10 Minutes
Ingredients:
- 1 pound (454 g) tiger shrimp
- 2 tablespoons olive oil
- ½ tablespoon old bay seasoning
- ¼ tablespoon smoked paprika
- ¼ teaspoon cayenne pepper
- A pinch of sea salt

Directions:
1. Toss all the ingredients in a large bowl until the shrimp are evenly coated.
2. Arrange the shrimp in the air fryer basket.
3. Put the air fryer basket on the baking pan and slide into Rack Position 2, select Air Fry, set temperature to 380ºF (193ºC), and set time to 10 minutes.
4. When cooking is complete, the shrimp should be pink and cooked through. Remove from the oven and serve hot.

220.Baked Buttery Shrimp

Servings: 4
Cooking Time: 15 Minutes
Ingredients:
- 1 lb shrimp, peel & deveined
- 2 tsp garlic powder
- 2 tsp dry mustard
- 2 tsp cumin

- 2 tsp paprika
- 2 tsp black pepper
- 4 tsp cayenne pepper
- 1/2 cup butter, melted
- 2 tsp onion powder
- 1 tsp dried oregano
- 1 tsp dried thyme
- 3 tsp salt

Directions:
1. Fit the Breville Smart oven with the rack in position
2. Add shrimp, butter, and remaining ingredients into the mixing bowl and toss well.
3. Transfer shrimp mixture into the baking pan.
4. Set to bake at 400 F for 20 minutes. After 5 minutes place the baking pan in the preheated oven.
5. Serve and enjoy.
- **Nutrition Info:** Calories 372 Fat 26.2 g Carbohydrates 7.5 g Sugar 1.3 g Protein 27.6 g Cholesterol 300 mg

221.Perfect Baked Cod

Servings: 4
Cooking Time: 15 Minutes
Ingredients:
- 4 cod fillets
- 1 tbsp olive oil
- 1 tsp dried parsley
- 2 tsp paprika
- 3/4 cup parmesan cheese, grated
- 1/4 tsp salt

Directions:
1. Fit the Breville Smart oven with the rack in position
2. In a shallow dish, mix parmesan cheese, paprika, parsley, and salt.
3. Brush fish fillets with oil and coat with parmesan cheese mixture.
4. Place coated fish fillets into the baking dish.
5. Set to bake at 400 F for 20 minutes. After 5 minutes place the baking dish in the preheated oven.
6. Serve and enjoy.

- **Nutrition Info:** Calories 160 Fat 8.1 g Carbohydrates 1.2 g Sugar 0.1 g Protein 21.7 g Cholesterol 56 mg

222.Spicy Lemon Garlic Tilapia

Servings: 2
Cooking Time: 15 Minutes
Ingredients:
- 4 tilapia fillets
- 1 lemon, cut into slices
- 1/2 tsp pepper
- 1/2 tsp chili powder
- 1 tsp garlic, minced
- 3 tbsp butter, melted
- 1 tbsp fresh lemon juice
- Salt

Directions:
1. Fit the Breville Smart oven with the rack in position
2. Place fish fillets into the baking dish.
3. Arrange lemon slices on top of fish fillets.
4. Mix together the remaining ingredients and pour over fish fillets.
5. Set to bake at 350 F for 20 minutes. After 5 minutes place the baking dish in the preheated oven.
6. Serve and enjoy.
- **Nutrition Info:** Calories 354 Fat 19.6 g Carbohydrates 4 g Sugar 1 g Protein 42.8 g Cholesterol 156 mg

223.Breaded Calamari With Lemon

Servings:4
Cooking Time: 12 Minutes
Ingredients:
- 2 large eggs
- 2 garlic cloves, minced
- ½ cup cornstarch
- 1 cup bread crumbs
- 1 pound (454 g) calamari rings
- Cooking spray
- 1 lemon, sliced

Directions:
1. In a small bowl, whisk the eggs with minced garlic. Place the cornstarch and bread crumbs into separate shallow dishes.
2. Dredge the calamari rings in the cornstarch, then dip in the egg mixture, shaking off any excess, finally roll them in the bread crumbs to coat well. Let the calamari rings sit for 10 minutes in the refrigerator.
3. Spritz the air fryer basket with cooking spray. Transfer the calamari rings to the pan.
4. Put the air fryer basket on the baking pan and slide into Rack Position 2, select Air Fry, set temperature to 390ºF (199ºC), and set time to 12 minutes.
5. Stir the calamari rings once halfway through the cooking time.
6. When cooking is complete, remove from the oven. Serve the calamari rings with the lemon slices sprinkled on top.

224.Coconut Chili Fish Curry

Servings:4
Cooking Time: 22 Minutes
Ingredients:
- 2 tablespoons sunflower oil, divided
- 1 pound (454 g) fish, chopped
- 1 ripe tomato, pureéd
- 2 red chilies, chopped
- 1 shallot, minced
- 1 garlic clove, minced
- 1 cup coconut milk
- 1 tablespoon coriander powder
- 1 teaspoon red curry paste
- ½ teaspoon fenugreek seeds
- Salt and white pepper, to taste

Directions:
1. Coat the air fryer basket with 1 tablespoon of sunflower oil. Place the fish in the basket.
2. Put the air fryer basket on the baking pan and slide into Rack Position 2, select Air Fry, set temperature to 380ºF (193ºC), and set time to 10 minutes.
3. Flip the fish halfway through the cooking time.
4. When cooking is complete, transfer the cooked fish to the baking pan greased with the remaining 1 tablespoon of sunflower oil. Stir in the remaining ingredients.
5. Put the air fryer basket on the baking pan and slide into Rack Position 2, select Air Fry, set temperature to 350ºF (180ºC), and set time to 12 minutes.

6. When cooking is complete, they should be heated through. Cool for 5 to 8 minutes before serving.

225. Herb Baked Catfish Fillets

Servings: 4
Cooking Time: 20 Minutes
Ingredients:
- 4 catfish fillets
- 1/2 tsp garlic powder
- 2 tbsp butter, melted
- 1 lemon juice
- 1/2 tsp pepper
- 1/2 tsp dried basil
- 1/2 tsp dried thyme
- 3/4 tsp paprika
- 1/2 tsp dried oregano
- 1 tsp salt

Directions:
1. Fit the Breville Smart oven with the rack in position
2. Place fish fillets into the baking pan.
3. Mix together garlic powder, pepper, basil, oregano, thyme, paprika, and salt and sprinkle over fish fillets.
4. Pour lemon juice and melted butter over fish fillets.
5. Set to bake at 350 F for 25 minutes. After 5 minutes place the baking pan in the preheated oven.
6. Serve and enjoy.
- **Nutrition Info:** Calories 274 Fat 18.1 g Carbohydrates 1.1 g Sugar 0.4 g Protein 25.2 g Cholesterol 90 mg

226. Seafood Mac N Cheese

Servings: 8
Cooking Time: 30 Minutes
Ingredients:
- Nonstick cooking spray
- 16 oz. macaroni
- 7 tbsp. butter, divided
- ¾ lb. medium shrimp, peel, devein, & cut in ½-inch pieces
- ½ cup Italian panko bread crumbs
- 1 cup onion, chopped fine
- 1 ½ tsp garlic, diced fine
- 1/3 cup flour
- 3 cups milk
- 1/8 tsp nutmeg
- ½ tsp Old Bay seasoning
- 1 tsp salt
- ¾ tsp pepper
- 1 1/3 cup Parmesan cheese, grated
- 1 1/3 cup Swiss cheese, grated
- 1 1/3 cup sharp cheddar cheese, grated
- ½ lb. lump crab meat, cooked

Directions:
1. Place wire rack in position 1 of the oven. Spray a 7x11-inch baking dish with cooking spray.
2. Cook macaroni according to package directions, shortening cooking time by 2 minutes. Drain and rinse with cold water.
3. Melt 1 tablespoon butter in a large skillet over med-high heat. Add shrimp and cook, stirring, until they turn pink. Remove from heat.
4. Melt remaining butter in a large saucepan over medium heat. Once melted, transfer 2 tablespoons to a small bowl and mix in bread crumbs.
5. Add onions and garlic to saucepan and cook, stirring, until they soften.
6. Whisk in flour and cook 1 minute, until smooth.
7. Whisk in milk until there are no lumps. Bring to a boil, reduce heat and simmer until thickened, whisking constantly.
8. Whisk in seasonings. Stir in cheese until melted and smooth. Fold in macaroni and seafood. Transfer to prepared dish. Sprinkle bread crumb mixture evenly over top.
9. Set oven to bake on 400°F for 25 minutes. After 5 minutes, place dish on the rack and bake 20 minutes, until topping is golden brown and sauce is bubbly. Let cool 5 minutes before serving.
- **Nutrition Info:** Calories 672, Total Fat 26g, Saturated Fat 15g, Total Carbs 68g, Net Carbs 61g, Protein 39g, Sugar 7g, Fiber 7g, Sodium 996mg, Potassium 921mg, Phosphorus 714mg

227. Salmon Fritters

Servings: x

Cooking Time:x

Ingredients:

- 2 tbsp. garam masala
- 1 lb. fileted Salmon
- 3 tsp ginger finely chopped
- 1-2 tbsp. fresh coriander leaves
- 2 or 3 green chilies finely chopped
- 1 ½ tbsp. lemon juice
- Salt and pepper to taste

Directions:

1. Mix the ingredients in a clean bowl.
2. Mold this mixture into round and flat French Cuisine Galettes.
3. Wet the French Cuisine Galettes slightly with water.
4. Pre heat the Breville smart oven at 160 degrees Fahrenheit for 5 minutes. Place the French Cuisine Galettes in the fry basket and let them cook for another 25 minutes at the same temperature. Keep rolling them over to get a uniform cook. Serve either with mint sauce or ketchup.

228.Air Fry Tuna Patties

Servings: 4

Cooking Time: 6 Minutes

Ingredients:

- 1 egg, lightly beaten
- 8 oz can tuna, drained
- 1/4 cup breadcrumbs
- 1 tbsp mustard
- 1/4 tsp garlic powder
- Pepper
- Salt

Directions:

1. Fit the Breville Smart oven with the rack in position 2.
2. Add all ingredients into the large bowl and mix until well combined.
3. Make four equal shapes of patties from the mixture and place in the air fryer basket then place an air fryer basket in the baking pan.
4. Place a baking pan on the oven rack. Set to air fry at 400 F for 6 minutes.
5. Serve and enjoy.

- **Nutrition Info:** Calories 122 Fat 2.7 g Carbohydrates 6.1 g Sugar 0.7 g Protein 17.5 g Cholesterol 58 mg

229.Buttery Crab Legs

Servings:4

Cooking Time: 15 Minutes

Ingredients:

- 3 pounds crab legs
- 1 cup butter, melted

Directions:

1. Preheat Breville on AirFry function to 380 F. Dip the crab legs in salted water and let stay for a few minutes. Drain, pat dry, and place the legs in the basket and press Start. Cook for 10 minutes. Pour the butter over crab legs and serve.

230.Spicy Lemon Cod

Servings: 2

Cooking Time: 10 Minutes

Ingredients:

- 1 lb cod fillets
- 1/4 tsp chili powder
- 1 tbsp fresh parsley, chopped
- 1 1/2 tbsp olive oil
- 1 tbsp fresh lemon juice
- 1/8 tsp cayenne pepper
- 1/4 tsp salt

Directions:

1. Fit the Breville Smart oven with the rack in position
2. Arrange fish fillets in a baking dish. Drizzle with oil and lemon juice.
3. Sprinkle with chili powder, salt, and cayenne pepper.
4. Set to bake at 400 F for 15 minutes. After 5 minutes place the baking dish in the preheated oven.
5. Garnish with parsley and serve.

- **Nutrition Info:** Calories 276 Fat 12.7 g Carbohydrates 0.5 g Sugar 0.2 g Protein 40.7 g Cholesterol 111 mg

231.Shrimp Momo's Recipe

Servings:x

Cooking Time:x

Ingredients:

- 1 ½ cup all-purpose flour
- ½ tsp. salt
- 5 tbsp. water
- For filling:
- 2 cups minced shrimp
- 2 tbsp. oil
- 2 tsp. ginger-garlic paste
- 2 tsp. soya sauce
- 2 tsp. vinegar

Directions:

1. Squeeze the dough and cover it with plastic wrap and set aside. Next, cook the ingredients for the filling and try to ensure that the shrimp is covered well with the sauce. Roll the dough and cut it into a square. Place the filling in the center.
2. Now, wrap the dough to cover the filling and pinch the edges together. Pre heat the Breville smart oven at 200° F for 5 minutes. Place the wontons in the fry basket and close it. Let them cook at the same temperature for another 20 minutes. Recommended sides are chili sauce or ketchup.

232.Spinach Scallops

Servings: 2
Cooking Time: 10 Minutes
Ingredients:

- 8 sea scallops
- 1 tbsp fresh basil, chopped
- 1 tbsp tomato paste
- 3/4 cup heavy cream
- 12 oz frozen spinach, thawed and drained
- 1 tsp garlic, minced
- 1/2 tsp pepper
- 1/2 tsp salt

Directions:

1. Fit the Breville Smart oven with the rack in position
2. Layer spinach in the baking dish.
3. Spray scallops with cooking spray and season with pepper and salt.
4. Place scallops on top of spinach.
5. In a small bowl, mix garlic, basil, tomato paste, whipping cream, pepper, and salt and pour over scallops and spinach.

6. Set to bake at 350 F for 15 minutes. After 5 minutes place the baking dish in the preheated oven.
7. Serve and enjoy.
- **Nutrition Info:** Calories 310 Fat 18.3 g Carbohydrates 12.6 g Sugar 1.7 g Protein 26.5 g Cholesterol 101 mg

233.Browned Shrimp Patties

Servings:4
Cooking Time: 12 Minutes
Ingredients:

- ½ pound (227 g) raw shrimp, shelled, deveined, and chopped finely
- 2 cups cooked sushi rice
- ¼ cup chopped red bell pepper
- ¼ cup chopped celery
- ¼ cup chopped green onion
- 2 teaspoons Worcestershire sauce
- ½ teaspoon salt
- ½ teaspoon garlic powder
- ½ teaspoon Old Bay seasoning
- ½ cup plain bread crumbs
- Cooking spray

Directions:

1. Put all the ingredients except the bread crumbs and oil in a large bowl and stir to incorporate.
2. Scoop out the shrimp mixture and shape into 8 equal-sized patties with your hands, no more than ½-inch thick. Roll the patties in the bread crumbs on a plate and spray both sides with cooking spray. Place the patties in the air fryer basket.
3. Put the air fryer basket on the baking pan and slide into Rack Position 2, select Air Fry, set temperature to 390ºF (199ºC), and set time to 12 minutes.
4. Flip the patties halfway through the cooking time.
5. When cooking is complete, the outside should be crispy brown. Divide the patties among four plates and serve warm.

234.Spicy Orange Shrimp

Servings:4
Cooking Time: 12 Minutes
Ingredients:

- $^1/_3$ cup orange juice
- 3 teaspoons minced garlic
- 1 teaspoon Old Bay seasoning
- ¼ to ½ teaspoon cayenne pepper
- 1 pound (454 g) medium shrimp, thawed, deveined, peeled, with tails off, and patted dry
- Cooking spray

Directions:

1. Stir together the orange juice, garlic, Old Bay seasoning, and cayenne pepper in a medium bowl. Add the shrimp to the bowl and toss to coat well.
2. Cover the bowl with plastic wrap and marinate in the refrigerator for 30 minutes.
3. Spritz the air fryer basket with cooking spray. Place the shrimp in the pan and spray with cooking spray.
4. Put the air fryer basket on the baking pan and slide into Rack Position 2, select Air Fry, set temperature to 400ºF (205ºC), and set time to 12 minutes.
5. Flip the shrimp halfway through the cooking time.
6. When cooked, the shrimp should be opaque and crisp. Remove from the oven and serve hot.

MEATLESS RECIPES

235. Lemony Brussels Sprouts And Tomatoes

Servings: 4
Cooking Time: 20 Minutes
Ingredients:
- 1 pound (454 g) Brussels sprouts, trimmed and halved
- 1 tablespoon extra-virgin olive oil
- Sea Salt and freshly ground black pepper, to taste
- ½ cup sun-dried tomatoes, chopped
- 2 tablespoons freshly squeezed lemon juice
- 1 teaspoon lemon zest

Directions:
1. Line the air fryer basket with aluminum foil.
2. Toss the Brussels sprouts with the olive oil in a large bowl. Sprinkle with salt and black pepper.
3. Spread the Brussels sprouts in a single layer in the basket.
4. Put the air fryer basket on the baking pan and slide into Rack Position 2, select Roast, set temperature to 400ºF (205ºC), and set time to 20 minutes.
5. When done, the Brussels sprouts should be caramelized. Remove from the oven to a serving bowl, along with the tomatoes, lemon juice, and lemon zest. Toss to combine. Serve immediately.

236. Sweet Baby Carrots

Servings: 4
Cooking Time: 20 Minutes
Ingredients:
- 1 pound baby carrots
- 1 tsp dried dill
- 1 tbsp olive oil
- 1 tbsp honey
- Salt and black pepper to taste

Directions:
1. Preheat your Breville Smart Oven to 300 F on Air Fry function. In a bowl, mix oil, carrots, and honey; gently stir to coat. Season with dill, pepper, and salt. Place the carrots in the cooking basket and fit in the baking tray; cook for 15 minutes, shaking once. Serve.

237. Macaroni Fried Baked Pastry

Servings: x
Cooking Time: x
Ingredients:
- 2 carrot sliced
- 2 cabbage sliced
- 2 tbsp. soya sauce
- 2 tsp. vinegar
- Some salt and pepper to taste
- 2 tbsp. olive oil
- ½ tsp. axiomata
- 1 cup all-purpose flour
- 2 tbsp. unsalted butter
- A pinch of salt to taste
- Take the amount of water sufficient enough to make a stiff dough
- 3 cups boiled macaroni
- 2 onion sliced
- 2 capsicum sliced
- 2 tbsp. ginger finely chopped
- 2 tbsp. garlic finely chopped
- 2 tbsp. green chilies finely chopped
- 2 tbsp. ginger-garlic paste

Directions:
1. Mix the dough for the outer covering and make it stiff and smooth. Leave it to rest in a container while making the filling. Cook the ingredients in a pan and stir them well to make a thick paste. Roll the paste out.
2. Roll the dough into balls and flatten them. Cut them in halves and add the filling. Use water to help you fold the edges to create the shape of a cone. Pre-heat the Breville smart oven for around 5 to 6 minutes at 300 Fahrenheit. Place all the samosas in the fry basket and close the basket properly. Keep the Breville smart oven at 200 degrees for another 20 to 25 minutes.
3. Around the halfway point, open the basket and turn the samosas over for uniform cooking. After this, fry at 250 degrees for around 10 minutes in order to give them the desired golden-brown color. Serve hot.

Recommended sides are tamarind or mint sauce.

238.Zucchini Parmesan Chips

Servings: 10
Cooking Time: 8 Minutes
Ingredients:
- ½ tsp. paprika
- ½ C. grated parmesan cheese
- ½ C. Italian breadcrumbs
- 1 lightly beaten egg
- 2 thinly sliced zucchinis

Directions:
1. Preparing the Ingredients. Use a very sharp knife or mandolin slicer to slice zucchini as thinly as you can. Pat off extra moisture.
2. Beat egg with a pinch of pepper and salt and a bit of water.
3. Combine paprika, cheese, and breadcrumbs in a bowl.
4. Dip slices of zucchini into the egg mixture and then into breadcrumb mixture. Press gently to coat.
5. Air Frying. With olive oil cooking spray, mist coated zucchini slices. Place into your Breville Smart air fryer oven in a single layer. Set temperature to 350°F, and set time to 8 minutes.
6. Sprinkle with salt and serve with salsa.
- **Nutrition Info:** CALORIES: 211; FAT: 16G; PROTEIN:8G; SUGAR:0G

239.Cornflakes French Toast

Servings:x
Cooking Time:x
Ingredients:
- 1 tsp. sugar for every 2 slices
- Crushed cornflakes
- Bread slices (brown or white)
- 1 egg white for every 2 slices

Directions:
1. Put two slices together and cut them along the diagonal.
2. In a bowl, whisk the egg whites and add some sugar.
3. Dip the bread triangles into this mixture and then coat them with the crushed cornflakes.

4. Pre heat the Breville smart oven at 180° C for 4 minutes. Place the coated bread triangles in the fry basket and close it. Let them cook at the same temperature for another 20 minutes at least. Halfway through the process, turn the triangles over so that you get a uniform cook. Serve these slices with chocolate sauce.

240.Tortellini With Veggies And Parmesan

Servings:4
Cooking Time: 16 Minutes
Ingredients:
- 8 ounces (227 g) sugar snap peas, trimmed
- ½ pound (227 g) asparagus, trimmed and cut into 1-inch pieces
- 2 teaspoons kosher salt or 1 teaspoon fine salt, divided
- 1 tablespoon extra-virgin olive oil
- 1½ cups water
- 1 (20-ounce / 340-g) package frozen cheese tortellini
- 2 garlic cloves, minced
- 1 cup heavy (whipping) cream
- 1 cup cherry tomatoes, halved
- ½ cup grated Parmesan cheese
- ¼ cup chopped fresh parsley or basil
- Add the peas and asparagus to a large bowl. Add ½ teaspoon of kosher salt and the olive oil and toss until well coated. Place the veggies in the baking pan.

Directions:
1. Slide the baking pan into Rack Position 1, select Convection Bake, set the temperature to 450ºF (235ºC), and set the time for 4 minutes.
2. Meanwhile, dissolve 1 teaspoon of kosher salt in the water.
3. Once cooking is complete, remove the pan from the oven and place the tortellini in the pan. Pour the salted water over the tortellini. Put the pan back to the oven.
4. Slide the baking pan into Rack Position 1, select Convection Bake, set temperature to 450ºF (235ºC), and set time for 7 minutes.
5. Meantime, stir together the garlic, heavy cream, and remaining ½ teaspoon of kosher salt in a small bowl.

6. Once cooking is complete, remove the pan from the oven. Blot off any remaining water with a paper towel. Gently stir the ingredients. Drizzle the cream over and top with the tomatoes.
7. Slide the baking pan into Rack Position 2, select Roast, set the temperature to 375ºF (190ºC), and set the time for 5 minutes.
8. After 4 minutes, remove from the oven.
9. Add the Parmesan cheese and stir until the cheese is melted
10. Serve topped with the parsley.

241.Mushroom Marinade Cutlet

Servings:x
Cooking Time:x
Ingredients:
- 2 cup fresh green coriander
- ½ cup mint leaves
- 4 tsp. fennel
- 2 tbsp. ginger-garlic paste
- 1 small onion
- 6-7 flakes garlic (optional)
- Salt to taste
- 2 cups sliced mushrooms
- 1 big capsicum (Cut this capsicum into big cubes)
- 1 onion (Cut it into quarters. Now separate the layers carefully.)
- 5 tbsp. gram flour
- A pinch of salt to taste
- 3 tbsp. lemon juice

Directions:
1. Take a clean and dry container. Put into it the coriander, mint, fennel, and ginger, onion/garlic, salt and lemon juice. Mix them.
2. Pour the mixture into a grinder and blend until you get a thick paste. Slit the mushroom almost till the end and leave them aside. Now stuff all the pieces with the paste and set aside. Take the sauce and add to it the gram flour and some salt. Mix them together properly. Rub this mixture all over the stuffed mushroom.
3. Now, to the leftover sauce, add the capsicum and onions. Apply the sauce generously on each of the pieces of capsicum and onion. Now take satay sticks

and arrange the cottage cheese pieces and vegetables on separate sticks.
4. Pre heat the Breville smart oven at 290 Fahrenheit for around 5 minutes. Open the basket. Arrange the satay sticks properly. Close the basket. Keep the sticks with the mushroom at 180 degrees for around half an hour while the sticks with the vegetables are to be kept at the same temperature for only 7 minutes. Turn the sticks in between so that one side does not get burnt and also to provide a uniform cook.

242.Korean Tempeh Steak With Broccoli

Servings: 4
Cooking Time: 15 Minutes + Marinating Time
Ingredients:
- 16 oz tempeh, cut into 1 cm thick pieces
- 1 pound broccoli, cut into florets
- ⅓ cup fermented soy sauce
- 2 tbsp sesame oil
- ⅓ cup sherry
- 1 tsp soy sauce
- 1 tsp white sugar
- 1 tsp cornstarch
- 1 tbsp olive oil
- 1 garlic clove, minced

Directions:
1. In a bowl, mix cornstarch, sherry, fermented soy sauce, sesame oil, soy sauce, sugar, and tempeh pieces. Marinate for 45 minutes.
2. Then, add in garlic, olive oil, and ginger. Place in the basket and fit in the baking tray; cook for 10 minutes at 390 F on Air Fry function, turning once halfway through. Serve.

243.Vegetable Au Gratin

Servings: 3
Cooking Time: 30 Minutes
Ingredients:
- 1 cup cubed eggplant
- ¼ cup chopped red pepper
- ¼ cup chopped green pepper
- ¼ cup chopped onion
- ⅓ cup chopped tomatoes
- 1 clove garlic, minced

- 1 tbsp sliced pimiento-stuffed olives
- 1 tsp capers
- ¼ tsp dried basil
- ¼ tsp dried marjoram
- Salt and black pepper to taste
- ¼ cup grated mozzarella cheese
- 1 tbsp breadcrumbs

Directions:

1. In a bowl, add eggplant, peppers, onion, tomatoes, olives, garlic, basil, marjoram, capers, salt, and black pepper. Lightly grease a baking tray with cooking spray. Add in the vegetable mixture and spread it evenly. Sprinkle mozzarella cheese on top and cover with breadcrumbs. Cook in your Breville Smart for 20 minutes on Bake function at 360 F. Serve.

244.Cheesy Frittata With Vegetables

Servings: 2
Cooking Time: 25 Minutes
Ingredients:

- 1 cup baby spinach
- ⅓ cup sliced mushrooms
- 1 zucchini, sliced with a 1-inch thickness
- 1 small red onion, sliced
- ¼ cup chopped chives
- ¼ lb asparagus, trimmed and sliced thinly
- 2 tsp olive oil
- 4 eggs, cracked into a bowl
- ⅓ cup milk
- Salt and black pepper to taste
- ⅓ cup grated Cheddar cheese
- ⅓ cup crumbled Feta cheese

Directions:

1. Preheat Breville Smart on Bake function to 320 F. Line a baking dish with parchment paper. Mix the beaten eggs with milk, salt, and pepper.
2. Heat olive oil in a skillet over medium heat add stir-fry asparagus, zucchini, onion, mushrooms, and baby spinach for 5 minutes. Pour the veggies into the baking dish and top with the egg mixture. Sprinkle with feta and cheddar cheeses. Cook for 15 minutes. Garnish with chives.

245.Mozzarella Eggplant Patties

Servings: 1
Cooking Time: 10 Minutes
Ingredients:

- 1 hamburger bun
- 1 eggplant, sliced
- 1 mozzarella slice, chopped
- 1 red onion cut into 3 rings
- 1 lettuce leaf
- ½ tbsp tomato sauce
- 1 pickle, sliced

Directions:

1. Preheat Breville Smart on Bake function to 330 F. Place the eggplant slices in a greased baking tray and cook for 6 minutes. Take out the tray and top the eggplant with mozzarella cheese and cook for 30 more seconds. Spread tomato sauce on one half of the bun. Place the lettuce leaf on top of the sauce. Place the cheesy eggplant on top of the lettuce. Top with onion rings and pickles and then with the other bun half to serve.

246.Rosemary Beets With Balsamic Glaze

Servings:2
Cooking Time: 10 Minutes
Ingredients:

- Beet:
- 2 beets, cubed
- 2 tablespoons olive oil
- 2 springs rosemary, chopped
- Salt and black pepper, to taste
- Balsamic Glaze:
- $^1/_3$ cup balsamic vinegar
- 1 tablespoon honey

Directions:

1. Combine the beets, olive oil, rosemary, salt, and pepper in a mixing bowl and toss until the beets are completely coated.
2. Place the beets in the air fryer basket.
3. Put the air fryer basket on the baking pan and slide into Rack Position 2, select Air Fry, set temperature to 400ºF (205ºC) and set time to 10 minutes.
4. Stir the vegetables halfway through.

5. When cooking is complete, the beets should be crisp and browned at the edges.
6. Meanwhile, make the balsamic glaze: Place the balsamic vinegar and honey in a small saucepan and bring to a boil over medium heat. When the sauce boils, reduce the heat to medium-low heat and simmer until the liquid is reduced by half.
7. When ready, remove the beets from the oven to a platter. Pour the balsamic glaze over the top and serve immediately.

247.Onion Rings

Servings: 4
Cooking Time: 10 Minutes
Ingredients:
- 1 large spanish onion
- 1/2 cup buttermilk
- 2 eggs, lightly beaten
- 3/4 cups unbleached all-purpose flour
- 3/4 cups panko bread crumbs
- 1/2 teaspoon baking powder
- 1/2 teaspoon Cayenne pepper, to taste
- Salt

Directions:
1. Preparing the Ingredients. Start by cutting your onion into 1/2 thick rings and separate. Smaller pieces can be discarded or saved for other recipes.
2. Beat the eggs in a large bowl and mix in the buttermilk, then set it aside.
3. In another bowl combine flour, pepper, bread crumbs, and baking powder.
4. Use a large spoon to dip a whole ring in the buttermilk, then pull it through the flour mix on both sides to completely coat the ring.
5. Air Frying. Cook about 8 rings at a time in your Breville Smart air fryer oven for 8-10 minutes at 360 degrees shaking half way through.
- **Nutrition Info:** CALORIES: 225; FAT: 3.8G; PROTEIN:19G; FIBER:2.4G

248.Garlic Toast With Cheese

Servings:x
Cooking Time:x
Ingredients:

- ¾ cup grated cheese
- 2 tsp. of oregano seasoning
- Some red chili flakes to sprinkle on top
- Take some French bread and cut it into slices
- 1 tbsp. olive oil (Optional)
- 2 tbsp. softened butter
- 4-5 flakes crushed garlic
- A pinch of salt to taste
- ½ tsp. black pepper powder

Directions:
1. Take a clean and dry container. Place all the ingredients mentioned under the heading "Garlic Butter" into it and mix properly to obtain garlic butter. On each slice of the French bread, spread some of this garlic butter. Sprinkle some cheese on top of the layer of butter. Pour some oil if wanted.
2. Sprinkle some chili flakes and some oregano.
3. Pre heat the Breville smart oven at 240 Fahrenheit for around 5 minutes. Open the fry basket and place the bread in it making sure that no two slices touch each other. Close the basket and continue to cook the bread at 160 degrees for another 10 minutes to toast the bread well.

249.Pizza

Servings:x
Cooking Time:x
Ingredients:
- 2 tomatoes that have been deseeded and chopped
- 1 tbsp. (optional) mushrooms/corns
- 2 tsp. pizza seasoning
- Some cottage cheese that has been cut into small cubes (optional)
- One pizza base
- Grated pizza cheese (mozzarella cheese preferably) for topping
- Use cooking oil for brushing and topping purposes
- ingredients for topping:
- 2 onions chopped
- 2 capsicums chopped

Directions:

1. Put the pizza base in a pre-heated Breville smart oven for around 5 minutes. (Pre heated to 340 Fahrenheit). Take out the base.
2. Pour some pizza sauce on top of the base at the center. Using a spoon spread the sauce over the base making sure that you leave some gap around the circumference. Grate some mozzarella cheese and sprinkle it over the sauce layer. Take all the vegetables mentioned in the ingredient list above and mix them in a bowl.
3. Add some oil and seasoning. Also add some salt and pepper according to taste. Mix them properly. Put this topping over the layer of cheese on the pizza. Now sprinkle some more grated cheese and pizza seasoning on top of this layer.
4. Pre heat the Breville smart oven at 250 Fahrenheit for around 5 minutes. Open the fry basket and place the pizza inside. Close the basket and keep the fryer at 170 degrees for another 10 minutes. If you feel that it is undercooked you may put it at the same temperature for another 2 minutes or so.

250.Crispy Veggies With Halloumi

Servings:2
Cooking Time: 14 Minutes
Ingredients:
- 2 zucchinis, cut into even chunks
- 1 large eggplant, peeled, cut into chunks
- 1 large carrot, cut into chunks
- 6 ounces (170 g) halloumi cheese, cubed
- 2 teaspoons olive oil
- Salt and black pepper, to taste
- 1 teaspoon dried mixed herbs

Directions:
1. Combine the zucchinis, eggplant, carrot, cheese, olive oil, salt, and pepper in a large bowl and toss to coat well.
2. Spread the mixture evenly in the air fryer basket.
3. Put the air fryer basket on the baking pan and slide into Rack Position 2, select Air Fry, set temperature to 340ºF (171ºC), and set time to 14 minutes.

4. Stir the mixture once during cooking.
5. When cooking is complete, they should be crispy and golden. Remove from the oven and serve topped with mixed herbs.

251.Garlicky Sesame Carrots

Servings:4 To 6
Cooking Time: 16 Minutes
Ingredients:
- 1 pound (454 g) baby carrots
- 1 tablespoon sesame oil
- ½ teaspoon dried dill
- Pinch salt
- Freshly ground black pepper, to taste
- 6 cloves garlic, peeled
- 3 tablespoons sesame seeds

Directions:
1. In a medium bowl, drizzle the baby carrots with the sesame oil. Sprinkle with the dill, salt, and pepper and toss to coat well.
2. Place the baby carrots in the air fryer basket.
3. Put the air fryer basket on the baking pan and slide into Rack Position 2, select Roast, set temperature to 380ºF (193ºC), and set time to 16 minutes.
4. After 8 minutes, remove from the oven and stir in the garlic. Return the pan to the oven and continue roasting for 8 minutes more.
5. When cooking is complete, the carrots should be lightly browned. Remove from the oven and serve sprinkled with the sesame seeds.

252.Tangy Tofu

Servings:2
Cooking Time: 30 Minutes
Ingredients:
- 6 oz extra firm tofu
- Black pepper to taste
- 1 tbsp vegetable broth
- 1 tbsp soy sauce
- ⅓ tsp dried oregano
- ⅓ tsp garlic powder
- ⅓ tsp dried basil
- ⅓ tsp onion powder

Directions:
1. Place the tofu on a cutting board, and cut it into 3 lengthwise slices with a knife. Line a

side of the cutting board with paper towels, place the tofu on it and cover with a paper towel.

2. Use your hands to press the tofu gently until as much liquid has been extracted from it. Remove the paper towels and chop the tofu into 8 cubes; set aside.

3. In another bowl, add soy sauce, broth, oregano, basil, garlic powder, onion powder, and black pepper; mix well. Pour the spice mixture over the tofu and stir to coat; marinate for 10 minutes.

4. Preheat Breville on AirFry function to 390 F. Arrange the tofu on the frying basket in a single layer and Press Start. Cook for 10 minutes. Remove to a plate and serve with green salad.

253.Burger Cutlet

Servings:x
Cooking Time:x
Ingredients:
- 1 tbsp. fresh coriander leaves. Chop them finely
- ¼ tsp. red chili powder
- ½ cup of boiled peas
- ¼ tsp. cumin powder
- 1 large potato boiled and mashed
- ½ cup breadcrumbs
- A pinch of salt to taste
- ¼ tsp. ginger finely chopped
- 1 green chili finely chopped
- 1 tsp. lemon juice
- ¼ tsp. dried mango powder

Directions:
1. Mix the ingredients together and ensure that the flavors are right. You will now make round cutlets with the mixture and roll them out well.

2. Pre heat the Breville smart oven at 250 Fahrenheit for 5 minutes. Open the basket of the Fryer and arrange the cutlets in the basket. Close it carefully. Keep the fryer at 150 degrees for around 10 or 12 minutes. In between the cooking process, turn the cutlets over to get a uniform cook. Serve hot with mint sauce.

254.Cottage Cheese French Cuisine Galette

Servings:x
Cooking Time:x
Ingredients:
- 1-2 tbsp. fresh coriander leaves
- 2 or 3 green chilies finely chopped
- 1 ½ tbsp. lemon juice
- Salt and pepper to taste
- 2 tbsp. garam masala
- 2 cups grated cottage cheese
- 1 ½ cup coarsely crushed peanuts
- 3 tsp. ginger finely chopped

Directions:
1. Mix the ingredients in a clean bowl.
2. Mold this mixture into round and flat French Cuisine Galettes.
3. Wet the French Cuisine Galettes slightly with water. Coat each French Cuisine Galette with the crushed peanuts.
4. Pre heat the Breville smart oven at 160 degrees Fahrenheit for 5 minutes. Place the French Cuisine Galettes in the fry basket and let them cook for another 25 minutes at the same temperature. Keep rolling them over to get a uniform cook. Serve either with mint sauce or ketchup.

255.Cheesy Asparagus And Potato Platter

Servings:5
Cooking Time: 26 Minutes
Ingredients:
- 4 medium potatoes, cut into wedges
- Cooking spray
- 1 bunch asparagus, trimmed
- 2 tablespoons olive oil
- Salt and pepper, to taste
- Cheese Sauce:
- ¼ cup crumbled cottage cheese
- ¼ cup buttermilk
- 1 tablespoon whole-grain mustard
- Salt and black pepper, to taste

Directions:
1. Spritz the air fryer basket with cooking spray.
2. Put the potatoes in the air fryer basket.
3. Put the air fryer basket on the baking pan and slide into Rack Position 2, select Roast,

set temperature to 400ºF (205ºC) and set time to 20 minutes.

4. Stir the potatoes halfway through.
5. When cooking is complete, the potatoes should be golden brown.
6. Remove the potatoes from the oven to a platter. Cover the potatoes with foil to keep warm. Set aside.
7. Place the asparagus in the air fryer basket and drizzle with the olive oil. Sprinkle with salt and pepper.
8. Put the air fryer basket on the baking pan and slide into Rack Position 2, select Roast, set temperature to 400ºF (205ºC) and set time to 6 minutes. Stir the asparagus halfway through.
9. When cooking is complete, the asparagus should be crispy.
10. Meanwhile, make the cheese sauce by stirring together the cottage cheese, buttermilk, and mustard in a small bowl. Season as needed with salt and pepper.
11. Transfer the asparagus to the platter of potatoes and drizzle with the cheese sauce. Serve immediately.

256.Cottage Cheese Best Homemade Croquette(2)

Servings:x
Cooking Time:x
Ingredients:

- 1 big capsicum (Cut this capsicum into big cubes)
- 1 onion (Cut it into quarters. Now separate the layers carefully.)
- 5 tbsp. gram flour
- A pinch of salt to taste
- 2 cup fresh green coriander
- ½ cup mint leaves
- 4 tsp. fennel
- 1 small onion
- 2 tbsp. ginger-garlic paste
- 6-7 garlic flakes (optional)
- 3 tbsp. lemon juice
- 2 cups cottage cheese cut into slightly thick and long pieces (similar to
- French fries)
- Salt

Directions:

1. Take a clean and dry container. Put into it the coriander, mint, fennel, and ginger, onion/garlic, salt and lemon juice. Mix them.
2. Pour the mixture into a grinder and blend until you get a thick paste. Now move on to the cottage cheese pieces.
3. Slit these pieces almost till the end and leave them aside. Now stuff all the pieces with the paste that was obtained from the previous step. Now leave the stuffed cottage cheese aside. Take the sauce and add to it the gram flour and some salt.
4. Mix them together properly. Rub this mixture all over the stuffed cottage cheese pieces. Now leave the cottage cheese aside. Now, to the leftover sauce, add the capsicum and onions. Apply the sauce generously on each of the pieces of capsicum and onion.
5. Now take satay sticks and arrange the cottage cheese pieces and vegetables on separate sticks. Pre heat the Breville smart oven at 290 Fahrenheit for around 5 minutes. Open the basket. Arrange the satay sticks properly. Close the basket.
6. Keep the sticks with the cottage cheese at 180 degrees for around half an hour while the sticks with the vegetables are to be kept at the same temperature for only 7 minutes. Turn the sticks in between so that one side does not get burnt and also to provide a uniform cook.

257.Okra Spicy Lemon Kebab

Servings:x
Cooking Time:x
Ingredients:

- 3 tsp. lemon juice
- 2 tsp. garam masala
- 4 tbsp. chopped coriander
- 3 tbsp. cream
- 3 tbsp. chopped capsicum
- 3 eggs
- 2 cups sliced okra
- 3 onions chopped
- 5 green chilies-roughly chopped
- 1 ½ tbsp. ginger paste

- 1 ½ tsp. garlic paste
- 1 ½ tsp. salt
- 2 ½ tbsp. white sesame seeds

Directions:

1. Grind the ingredients except for the egg and form a smooth paste. Coat the okra in the paste. Now, beat the eggs and add a little salt to it.
2. Dip the coated vegetables in the egg mixture and then transfer to the sesame seeds and coat the okra well. Place the vegetables on a stick.
3. Pre heat the Breville smart oven at 160 degrees Fahrenheit for around 5 minutes. Place the sticks in the basket and let them cook for another 25 minutes at the same temperature. Turn the sticks over in between the cooking process to get a uniform cook.

258.Roasted Butternut Squash With Maple Syrup

Servings:4
Cooking Time: 30 Minutes
Ingredients:

- 1 lb butternut squash
- 1 tsp dried rosemary
- 2 tbsp maple syrup
- Salt to taste

Directions:

1. Place the squash on a cutting board and peel. Cut in half and remove the seeds and pulp. Slice into wedges and season with salt. Spray with cooking spray and sprinkle with rosemary.
2. Preheat Breville on AirFry function to 350 F. Transfer the wedges to the greased basket without overlapping. Press Start and cook for 20 minutes. Serve drizzled with maple syrup.

259.Potato Fries With Ketchup

Servings:2
Cooking Time: 20 Minutes
Ingredients:

- 2 potatoes
- 1 tbsp ketchup
- 2 tbsp olive oil

- Salt and black pepper to taste

Directions:

1. Use a spiralizer to spiralize the potatoes. In a bowl, mix olive oil, salt, and pepper. Drizzle the potatoes with the oil mixture. Place them in the basket and press Start. Cook for 15 minutes on AirFry function at 360 F. Serve with ketchup or mayonnaise.

260.Vegetarian Meatballs

Servings:3
Cooking Time: 18 Minutes
Ingredients:

- ½ cup grated carrots
- ½ cup sweet onions
- 2 tablespoons olive oil
- 1 cup rolled oats
- ½ cup roasted cashews
- 2 cups cooked chickpeas
- Juice of 1 lemon
- 2 tablespoons soy sauce
- 1 tablespoon flax meal
- 1 teaspoon garlic powder
- 1 teaspoon cumin
- ½ teaspoon turmeric

Directions:

1. Mix the carrots, onions, and olive oil in the baking pan and stir to combine.
2. Slide the baking pan into Rack Position 2, select Roast, set temperature to 350ºF (180ºC) and set time to 6 minutes.
3. Stir the vegetables halfway through.
4. When cooking is complete, the vegetables should be tender.
5. Meanwhile, put the oats and cashews in a food processor or blender and pulse until coarsely ground. Transfer the mixture to a large bowl. Add the chickpeas, lemon juice, and soy sauce to the food processor and pulse until smooth. Transfer the chickpea mixture to the bowl of oat and cashew mixture.
6. Remove the carrots and onions from the oven to the bowl of chickpea mixture. Add the flax meal, garlic powder, cumin, and turmeric and stir to incorporate.
7. Scoop tablespoon-sized portions of the veggie mixture and roll them into balls with

your hands. Transfer the balls to the air fryer basket.

8. Increase the temperature to 370ºF (188ºC) and set time to 12 minutes on Bake. Flip the balls halfway through the cooking time.
9. When cooking is complete, the balls should be golden brown.
10. Serve warm.

261.Chili Sweet Potato Fries

Servings:4
Cooking Time: 30 Minutes
Ingredients:
- ½ tsp salt
- ½ tsp garlic powder
- ½ tsp chili powder
- ¼ tsp ground cumin
- 3 tbsp olive oil
- 3 sweet potatoes, cut into thick strips

Directions:
1. In a bowl, mix salt, garlic powder, chili powder, and cumin, and whisk in oil. Coat in the potato strips and arrange them on the basket, without overcrowding. Press Start and cook for 20-25 minutes at 380 F on AirFry function or until crispy. Serve hot.

262.Asparagus French Cuisine Galette

Servings:x
Cooking Time:x
Ingredients:
- 1 ½ tbsp. lemon juice
- Salt and pepper to taste
- 2 cups minced asparagus
- 3 tsp. ginger finely chopped
- 1-2 tbsp. fresh coriander leaves
- 2 or 3 green chilies finely chopped

Directions:
1. Mix the ingredients in a clean bowl.
2. Mold this mixture into round and flat French Cuisine Galettes.
3. Wet the French Cuisine Galettes slightly with water.
4. Pre heat the Breville smart oven at 160 degrees Fahrenheit for 5 minutes. Place the French Cuisine Galettes in the fry basket and let them cook for another 25 minutes at the same temperature. Keep rolling them

over to get a uniform cook. Serve either with mint sauce or ketchup.

263.Potato Fried Baked Pastry

Servings:x
Cooking Time:x
Ingredients:
- 1 tsp. powdered ginger
- 1 or 2 green chilies that are finely chopped or mashed
- ½ tsp. cumin
- 1 tsp. coarsely crushed coriander
- 1 dry red chili broken into pieces
- A small amount of salt (to taste)
- 2 tbsp. unsalted butter
- 1 ½ cup all-purpose flour
- A pinch of salt to taste
- Add as much water as required to make the dough stiff and firm
- 2-3 big potatoes boiled and mashed
- ¼ cup boiled peas
- ½ tsp. dried mango powder
- ½ tsp. red chili power.
- 1-2 tbsp. coriander.

Directions:
1. Mix the dough for the outer covering and make it stiff and smooth. Leave it to rest in a container while making the filling. Cook the ingredients in a pan and stir them well to make a thick paste. Roll the paste out.
2. Roll the dough into balls and flatten them. Cut them in halves and add the filling. Use water to help you fold the edges to create the shape of a cone. Pre-heat the Breville smart oven for around 5 to 6 minutes at 300 Fahrenheit.
3. Place all the samosas in the fry basket and close the basket properly. Keep the Breville smart oven at 200 degrees for another 20 to 25 minutes. Around the halfway point, open the basket and turn the samosas over for uniform cooking. After this, fry at 250 degrees for around 10 minutes in order to give them the desired golden-brown color. Serve hot. Recommended sides are tamarind or mint sauce.

264.Tomato & Feta Bites With Pine Nuts

Servings:2
Cooking Time: 25 Minutes
Ingredients:

- 1 heirloom tomato, sliced
- 1 (4- oz) block Feta cheese, sliced
- 1 small red onion, thinly sliced
- 1 clove garlic
- 2 tsp + ¼ cup olive oil
- 1 ½ tbsp toasted pine nuts
- ¼ cup fresh parsley, chopped
- ¼ cup grated Parmesan cheese
- ¼ cup chopped basil

Directions:

1. Add basil, pine nuts, garlic, and salt to a food processor. Process while slowly adding ¼ cup of olive oil. Once finished, pour basil pesto into a bowl and refrigerate for 30 minutes.
2. Preheat Breville oven on AirFry function to 390 F. Spread some pesto on each slice of tomato.
3. Top with feta cheese and onion and drizzle with the remaining olive oil. Place in the frying basket and press Start. Cook for 12 minutes. Top with the remaining pesto and serve.

265.Cheese And Mushroom Spicy Lemon Kebab

Servings:x
Cooking Time:x
Ingredients:

- 1-2 tbsp. all-purpose flour for coating purposes
- 1-2 tbsp. mint
- 1 cup molten cheese
- 1 onion that has been finely chopped
- ½ cup milk
- 2 cups sliced mushrooms
- 1-2 green chilies chopped finely
- ¼ tsp. red chili powder
- A pinch of salt to taste
- ½ tsp. dried mango powder
- ¼ tsp. black salt

Directions:

1. Take the mushroom slices and add the grated ginger and the cut green chilies. Grind this mixture until it becomes a thick paste.
2. Keep adding water as and when required. Now add the onions, mint, the breadcrumbs and all the various masalas required. Mix this well until you get a soft dough. Now take small balls of this mixture (about the size of a lemon) and mold them into the shape of flat and round kebabs. Here is where the milk comes into play.
3. Pour a very small amount of milk onto each kebab to wet it. Now roll the kebab in the dry breadcrumbs. Pre heat the Breville smart oven for 5 minutes at 300 Fahrenheit. Take out the basket. Arrange the kebabs in the basket leaving gaps between them so that no two kebabs are touching each other. Keep the fryer at 340 Fahrenheit for around half an hour.
4. Half way through the cooking process, turn the kebabs over so that they can be cooked properly. Recommended sides for this dish are mint sauce, tomato ketchup or yoghurt sauce.

266.Herbed Broccoli With Cheese

Servings:4
Cooking Time: 18 Minutes
Ingredients:

- 1 large-sized head broccoli, stemmed and cut into small florets
- 2½ tablespoons canola oil
- 2 teaspoons dried basil
- 2 teaspoons dried rosemary
- Salt and ground black pepper, to taste
- $1/3$ cup grated yellow cheese

Directions:

1. Bring a pot of lightly salted water to a boil. Add the broccoli florets to the boiling water and let boil for about 3 minutes.
2. Drain the broccoli florets well and transfer to a large bowl. Add the canola oil, basil, rosemary, salt, and black pepper to the bowl and toss until the broccoli is fully coated. Place the broccoli in the air fryer basket.

3. Put the air fryer basket on the baking pan and slide into Rack Position 2, select Air Fry, set temperature to 390ºF (199ºC), and set time to 15 minutes.
4. Stir the broccoli halfway through the cooking time.
5. When cooking is complete, the broccoli should be crisp. Serve the broccoli warm with grated cheese sprinkled on top.

267.Herby Tofu

Servings: 2
Cooking Time: 30 Minutes
Ingredients:
- 6 oz extra firm tofu
- Black pepper to taste
- 1 tbsp vegetable broth
- 1 tbsp soy sauce
- ⅓ tsp dried oregano
- ⅓ tsp garlic powder
- ⅓ tsp dried basil
- ⅓ tsp onion powder

Directions:
1. Place the tofu on a cutting board and cut it into 3 lengthwise slices with a knife. Line a side of the cutting board with paper towels, place the tofu on it, and cover with a paper towel. Use your hands to press the tofu gently until as much liquid has been extracted from it. Chop the tofu into 8 cubes; set aside.
2. In another bowl, add the soy sauce, vegetable broth, oregano, basil, garlic powder, onion powder, and black pepper and mix well with a spoon. Rub the spice mixture on the tofu. Let it marinate for 10 minutes.
3. Preheat Breville Smart on Air Fry function to 390 F. Place the tofu in the fryer's basket in a single layer and fit in the baking tray. Cook for 10 minutes, flipping it at the 6-minute mark. Remove to a plate and serve with green salad.

268.Apricot Spicy Lemon Kebab

Servings:x
Cooking Time:x
Ingredients:

- 3 tsp. lemon juice
- 2 tsp. garam masala
- 3 eggs
- 2 ½ tbsp. white sesame seeds
- 2 cups fresh apricots
- 3 onions chopped
- 5 green chilies-roughly chopped
- 1 ½ tbsp. ginger paste
- 1 ½ tsp. garlic paste
- 1 ½ tsp. salt

Directions:
1. Grind the ingredients except for the egg and form a smooth paste. Coat the apricots in the paste. Now, beat the eggs and add a little salt to it.
2. Dip the coated apricots in the egg mixture and then transfer to the sesame seeds and coat the apricots well. Place the vegetables on a stick.
3. Pre heat the Breville smart oven at 160 degrees Fahrenheit for around 5 minutes. Place the sticks in the basket and let them cook for another 25 minutes at the same temperature. Turn the sticks over in between the cooking process to get a uniform cook.

269.Cheesy Cabbage Wedges

Servings: 4
Cooking Time: 25 Minutes
Ingredients:
- ½ head cabbage, cut into wedges
- 2 cups Parmesan cheese, chopped
- 4 tbsp melted butter
- Salt and black pepper to taste
- ½ cup blue cheese sauce

Directions:
1. Brush the cabbage wedges with butter and coat with mozzarella cheese. Place the coated wedges in the greased basket and fit in the baking tray; cook for 20 minutes at 380 F on Air Fry setting. Serve with blue cheese sauce.

270.Stuffed Peppers With Beans And Rice

Servings:4
Cooking Time: 18 Minutes
Ingredients:

- 4 medium red, green, or yellow bell peppers, halved and deseeded
- 4 tablespoons extra-virgin olive oil, divided
- ½ teaspoon kosher salt, divided
- 1 (15-ounce / 425-g) can chickpeas
- 1½ cups cooked white rice
- ½ cup diced roasted red peppers
- ¼ cup chopped parsley
- ½ small onion, finely chopped
- 3 garlic cloves, minced
- ½ teaspoon cumin
- ¼ teaspoon freshly ground black pepper
- ¾ cup panko bread crumbs

Directions:
1. Brush the peppers inside and out with 1 tablespoon of olive oil. Season the insides with ¼ teaspoon of kosher salt. Arrange the peppers in the air fryer basket, cut side up.
2. Place the chickpeas with their liquid into a large bowl. Lightly mash the beans with a potato masher. Sprinkle with the remaining ¼ teaspoon of kosher salt and 1 tablespoon of olive oil. Add the rice, red peppers, parsley, onion, garlic, cumin, and black pepper to the bowl and stir to incorporate.
3. Divide the mixture among the bell pepper halves.
4. Stir together the remaining 2 tablespoons of olive oil and panko in a small bowl. Top the pepper halves with the panko mixture.
5. Put the air fryer basket on the baking pan and slide into Rack Position 2, select Roast, set temperature to 375ºF (190ºC), and set time to 18 minutes.
6. When done, the peppers should be slightly wrinkled, and the panko should be golden brown.
7. Remove from the oven and serve on a plate.

271.Cottage Cheese And Mushroom Mexican Burritos

Servings:x
Cooking Time:x
Ingredients:
- ½ cup mushrooms thinly sliced
- 1 cup cottage cheese cut in too long and slightly thick Oregano Fingers
- A pinch of salt to taste
- ½ tsp. red chili flakes
- 1 tsp. freshly ground peppercorns
- ½ cup pickled jalapenos
- 1-2 lettuce leaves shredded.
- ½ cup red kidney beans (soaked overnight)
- ½ small onion chopped
- 1 tbsp. olive oil
- 2 tbsp. tomato puree
- ¼ tsp. red chili powder
- 1 tsp. of salt to taste
- 4-5 flour tortillas
- 1 or 2 spring onions chopped finely. Also cut the greens.
- Take one tomato. Remove the seeds and chop it into small pieces.
- 1 green chili chopped.
- 1 cup of cheddar cheese grated.
- 1 cup boiled rice (not necessary).
- A few flour tortillas to put the filing in.

Directions:
1. Cook the beans along with the onion and garlic and mash them finely.
2. Now, make the sauce you will need for the burrito. Ensure that you create a slightly thick sauce.
3. For the filling, you will need to cook the ingredients well in a pan and ensure that the vegetables have browned on the outside.
4. To make the salad, toss the ingredients together. Place the tortilla and add a layer of sauce, followed by the beans and the filling at the center. Before you roll it, you will need to place the salad on top of the filling.
5. Pre-heat the Breville smart oven for around 5 minutes at 200 Fahrenheit. Open the fry basket and keep the burritos inside. Close the basket properly. Let the Air
6. Fryer remain at 200 Fahrenheit for another 15 minutes or so. Halfway through, remove the basket and turn all the burritos over in order to get a uniform cook.

272.Pumpkin French Cuisine Galette

Servings:x
Cooking Time:x
Ingredients:
- 2 or 3 green chilies finely chopped
- 1 ½ tbsp. lemon juice

- Salt and pepper to taste
- 2 tbsp. garam masala
- 1 cup sliced pumpkin
- 3 tsp. ginger finely chopped
- 1-2 tbsp. fresh coriander leaves

Directions:
1. Mix the ingredients in a clean bowl.
2. Mold this mixture into round and flat French Cuisine Galettes.
3. Wet the French Cuisine Galettes slightly with water.
4. Pre heat the Breville smart oven at 160 degrees Fahrenheit for 5 minutes. Place the French Cuisine Galettes in the fry basket and let them cook for another 25 minutes at the same temperature. Keep rolling them over to get a uniform cook. Serve either with mint sauce or ketchup.

273.Feta & Scallion Triangles

Servings:4
Cooking Time: 20 Minutes

Ingredients:
- 4 oz feta cheese, crumbled
- 2 sheets filo pastry
- 1 egg yolk, beaten
- 2 tbsp fresh parsley, finely chopped
- 1 scallion, finely chopped
- 2 tbsp olive oil
- Salt and black pepper to taste

Directions:
1. In a bowl, mix the yolk with the cheese, parsley, and scallion. Season with salt and black pepper. Cut each filo sheet in 3 strips. Put a teaspoon of the feta mixture on the bottom. Roll the strip in a spinning spiral way until the filling of the inside mixture is completely wrapped in a triangle.
2. Preheat Breville on Bake function to 360 F. Brush the surface of filo with olive oil. Place up to 5 triangles in the oven and press Start. Cook for 5 minutes. Lower the temperature to 330 F, cook for 3 more minutes or until golden brown.

SNACKS AND DESSERTS RECIPES

274.Bacon Cheese Jalapeno Poppers

Servings: 5
Cooking Time: 5 Minutes
Ingredients:
- 10 fresh jalapeno peppers, cut in half and remove seeds
- 1/4 cup cheddar cheese, shredded
- 5 oz cream cheese, softened
- ¼ tsp paprika
- 2 bacon slices, cooked and crumbled

Directions:
1. Fit the Breville Smart oven with the rack in position 2.
2. In a bowl, mix bacon, cream cheese, paprika and cheddar cheese.
3. Stuff cheese mixture into each jalapeno.
4. Place stuffed jalapeno halved in air fryer basket then place air fryer basket in baking pan.
5. Place a baking pan on the oven rack. Set to air fry at 370 F for 5 minutes.
6. Serve and enjoy.
- **Nutrition Info:** Calories 176 Fat 15.7 g Carbohydrates 3.2 g Sugar 1 g Protein 6.2 g Cholesterol 47 mg

275.Easy Blackberry Cobbler

Servings:6
Cooking Time: 20 To 25 Minutes
Ingredients:
- 3 cups fresh or frozen blackberries
- 1¾ cups sugar, divided
- 1 teaspoon vanilla extract
- 8 tablespoons (1 stick) butter, melted
- 1 cup self-rising flour
- Cooking spray

Directions:
1. Spritz the baking pan with cooking spray.
2. Mix the blackberries, 1 cup of sugar, and vanilla in a medium bowl and stir to combine.
3. Stir together the melted butter, remaining sugar, and flour in a separate medium bowl.
4. Spread the blackberry mixture evenly in the prepared pan and top with the butter mixture.

5. Slide the baking pan into Rack Position 1, select Convection Bake, set temperature to 350ºF (180ºC), and set time to 25 minutes.
6. After about 20 minutes, check if the cobbler has a golden crust and you can't see any batter bubbling while it cooks. If needed, bake for another 5 minutes.
7. Remove from the oven and place on a wire rack to cool to room temperature. Serve immediately.

276.Cheesy Spinach Dip

Servings: 12
Cooking Time: 20 Minutes
Ingredients:
- 3 oz frozen spinach, defrosted & chopped
- 1 cup sour cream
- 1 tsp garlic salt
- 2 cups cheddar cheese, shredded
- 8 oz cream cheese

Directions:
1. Fit the Breville Smart oven with the rack in position
2. Add all ingredients into the mixing bowl and mix well.
3. Transfer mixture into the baking dish.
4. Set to bake at 350 F for 25 minutes. After 5 minutes place the baking dish in the preheated oven.
5. Serve and enjoy.
- **Nutrition Info:** Calories 185 Fat 16.9 g Carbohydrates 2 g Sugar 0.3 g Protein 7 g Cholesterol 49 mg

277.Easy Bacon Jalapeno Poppers

Servings: 10
Cooking Time: 8 Minutes
Ingredients:
- 10 jalapeno peppers, cut in half and remove seeds
- 1/3 cup cream cheese, softened
- 1/4 tsp paprika
- 1/4 tsp chili powder
- 5 bacon strips, cut in half

Directions:
1. Fit the Breville Smart oven with the rack in position 2.

2. In a small bowl, mix cream cheese, paprika, chili powder, and bacon and stuff in each jalapeno half.
3. Place jalapeno half in the air fryer basket then place an air fryer basket in the baking pan.
4. Place a baking pan on the oven rack. Set to air fry at 370 F for 8 minutes.
5. Serve and enjoy.
- **Nutrition Info:** Calories 83 Fat 7.4 g Carbohydrates 1.3 g Sugar 0.5 g Protein 2.8 g Cholesterol 9 mg

278.Roasted Grapes With Yogurt

Servings:6
Cooking Time: 10 Minutes
Ingredients:
- 2 cups seedless red grapes, rinsed and patted dry
- 1 tablespoon apple cider vinegar
- 1 tablespoon honey
- 1 cup low-fat Greek yogurt
- 2 tablespoons 2 percent milk
- 2 tablespoons minced fresh basil

Directions:
1. Spread the red grapes in the baking pan and drizzle with the cider vinegar and honey. Lightly toss to coat.
2. Slide the baking pan into Rack Position 2, select Roast, set temperature to 380ºF (193ºC) and set time to 10 minutes.
3. When cooking is complete, the grapes will be wilted but still soft. Remove from the oven.
4. In a medium bowl, whisk together the yogurt and milk. Gently fold in the grapes and basil.
5. Serve immediately.

279.Perfectly Puffy Coconut Cookies

Servings: 12
Cooking Time: 15 Minutes
Ingredients:
- 1 cup butter, melted
- 1 ¾ cups granulated swerve
- 3 eggs
- 2 tablespoons coconut milk
- 1 teaspoon coconut extract
- 1 teaspoon vanilla extract
- 1 cup coconut flour
- 1 ¼ cups almond flour
- 1/2 teaspoon baking powder
- 1/2 teaspoon baking soda
- 1/2 teaspoon fine table salt
- 1/2 cups coconut chips, unsweetened

Directions:
1. Begin by preheating your Air Fryer to 350 degrees F.
2. In the bowl of an electric mixer, beat the butter and swerve until well combined. Now, add the eggs one at a time, and mix well; add the coconut milk, coconut extract, and vanilla; beat until creamy and uniform.
3. Mix the flour with baking powder, baking soda, and salt. Then, stir the flour mixture into the butter mixture and stir until everything is well incorporated.
4. Finally, fold in the coconut chips and mix again. Scoop out 1 tablespoon size balls of the batter on a cookie pan, leaving 2 inches between each cookie.
5. Bake for 10 minutes or until golden brown, rotating the pan once or twice through the cooking time. Let your cookies cool on wire racks.
- **Nutrition Info:** 304 Calories; 17g Fat; 32g Carbs; 3g Protein; 16g Sugars; 2g Fiber

280.Banana Clafouti

Servings:x
Cooking Time:x
Ingredients:
- 1 tsp vanilla extract
- 2 Tbsp butter, melted
- ¼ tsp salt
- ½ cup all-purpose flour
- 2 bananas, peeled and thinly sliced
- 2 tsp fresh lemon juice
- 1 cup whole milk
- ¼ cup whipping cream
- 3 eggs
- ½ cup granulated sugar

Directions:
1. Preheat the oven to 350°F.
2. Whisk together milk, cream, eggs, sugar, extract, butter and salt.

3. Add the flour and whisk gently until incorporated.
4. Place sliced bananas in a bowl with lemon juice.
5. Lightly grease Breville smart oven and heat in oven for 5 minutes. Remove and pour in batter.
6. Scatter bananas over batter and bake until golden and puffed, about 35 minutes.

281.Baked Almonds

Servings: 6
Cooking Time: 20 Minutes
Ingredients:
- 1 1/2 cups raw almonds
- 1/2 tsp cayenne
- 1/4 tsp onion powder
- 1/4 tsp dried basil
- 2 tbsp butter, melted
- 1/2 tsp garlic powder
- 1/2 tsp cumin
- 1 1/2 tsp chili powder
- 1/2 tsp sea salt

Directions:
1. Fit the Breville Smart oven with the rack in position
2. Add almonds and remaining ingredients into the mixing bowl and toss well.
3. Spread almonds in baking pan.
4. Set to bake at 350 F for 25 minutes. After 5 minutes place the baking pan in the preheated oven.
5. Serve and enjoy.
- **Nutrition Info:** Calories 176 Fat 15.9 g Carbohydrates 5.9 g Sugar 1.2 g Protein 5.2 g Cholesterol 10 mg

282.Baked Cream

Servings:x
Cooking Time:x
Ingredients:
- 1 cup fresh blueberries
- 1 cup blackberries
- Handful of mint leaves
- 3 tsp. sugar
- 2 cups condensed milk
- 2 cups fresh cream
- 1 cup fresh strawberries

- 4 tsp. water

Directions:
1. Blend the cream and add the milk to it. Whisk the ingredients well together and transfer this mixture into small baking bowls ensuring you do not overfill the bowls.
2. Preheat the fryer to 300 Fahrenheit for five minutes. You will need to place the bowls in the basket and cover it. Cook it for fifteen minutes. When you shake the bowls, the mixture should just shake but not break. Leave it in the refrigerator to set and then arrange the fruits, garnish and serve.

283.Apple Cake

Servings: 12
Cooking Time: 45 Minutes
Ingredients:
- 2 cups apples, peeled and chopped
- 1/4 cup sugar
- 1/4 cup butter, melted
- 12 oz apple juice
- 3 cups all-purpose flour
- 3 tsp baking powder
- 1 1/2 tbsp ground cinnamon
- 1 tsp Salt

Directions:
1. Fit the Breville Smart oven with the rack in position
2. In a large bowl, mix together flour, salt, sugar, cinnamon, and baking powder.
3. Add melted butter and apple juice and mix until well combined.
4. Add apples and fold well.
5. Pour batter into the greased baking dish.
6. Set to bake at 350 F for 45 minutes. After 5 minutes place the baking dish in the preheated oven.
7. Serve and enjoy.
- **Nutrition Info:** Calories 200 Fat 4 g Carbohydrates 38 g Sugar 11 g Protein 3 g Cholesterol 10 mg

284.Spiced Apple Chips

Servings:4
Cooking Time: 10 Minutes
Ingredients:

- 4 medium apples (any type will work), cored and thinly sliced
- ¼ teaspoon nutmeg
- ¼ teaspoon cinnamon
- Cooking spray

Directions:

1. Place the apple slices in a large bowl and sprinkle the spices on top. Toss to coat.
2. Put the apple slices in the air fryer basket in a single layer and spray them with cooking spray.
3. Put the air fryer basket on the baking pan and slide into Rack Position 2, select Air Fry, set temperature to 360ºF (182ºC), and set time to 10 minutes.
4. Stir the apple slices halfway through.
5. When cooking is complete, the apple chips should be crispy. Transfer the apple chips to a paper towel-lined plate and rest for 5 minutes before serving.

285.Baked Plums

Servings: 6
Cooking Time: 20 Minutes
Ingredients:

- 6 plums, cut into wedges
- 1 teaspoon ginger, ground
- ½ teaspoon cinnamon powder
- Zest of 1 lemon, grated
- 2 tablespoons water
- 10 drops stevia

Directions:

1. In a pan that fits the air fryer, combine the plums with the rest of the ingredients, toss gently, put the pan in the air fryer and cook at 360 degrees F for 20 minutes.
2. Serve cold.
- **Nutrition Info:** calories 170, fat 5, fiber 1, carbs 3, protein 5

286.Chocolate Chip Pan Cookie

Servings: 4
Cooking Time: 15 Minutes
Ingredients:

- ½ cup blanched finely ground almond flour.
- 1 large egg.
- ¼ cup powdered erythritol
- 2 tbsp. unsalted butter; softened.

- 2 tbsp. low-carb, sugar-free chocolate chips
- ½ tsp. unflavored gelatin
- ½ tsp. baking powder.
- ½ tsp. vanilla extract.

Directions:

1. Take a large bowl, mix almond flour and erythritol. Stir in butter, egg and gelatin until combined.
2. Stir in baking powder and vanilla and then fold in chocolate chips
3. Pour batter into 6-inch round baking pan. Place pan into the air fryer basket.
4. Adjust the temperature to 300 Degrees F and set the timer for 7 minutes
5. When fully cooked, the top will be golden brown and a toothpick inserted in center will come out clean. Let cool at least 10 minutes.
- **Nutrition Info:** Calories: 188; Protein: 5.6g; Fiber: 2.0g; Fat: 15.7g; Carbs: 16.8g

287.Fudge Pie

Servings:8
Cooking Time: 26 Minutes
Ingredients:

- 1½ cups sugar
- ½ cup self-rising flour
- $^1/_3$ cup unsweetened cocoa powder
- 3 large eggs, beaten
- 12 tablespoons (1½ sticks) butter, melted
- 1½ teaspoons vanilla extract
- 1 (9-inch) unbaked pie crust
- ¼ cup confectioners' sugar (optional)

Directions:

1. Thoroughly combine the sugar, flour, and cocoa powder in a medium bowl. Add the beaten eggs and butter and whisk to combine. Stir in the vanilla.
2. Pour the prepared filling into the pie crust and transfer to the baking pan.
3. Slide the baking pan into Rack Position 1, select Convection Bake, set temperature to 350ºF (180ºC), and set time to 26 minutes.
4. When cooking is complete, the pie should be set.
5. Allow the pie to cool for 5 minutes. Sprinkle with the confectioners' sugar, if desired. Serve warm.

288. Yummy Scalloped Pineapple

Servings: 6
Cooking Time: 35 Minutes
Ingredients:
- 3 eggs, lightly beaten
- 8 oz can crushed pineapple, un-drained
- 2 cups of sugar
- 4 cups of bread cubes
- 1/4 cup milk
- 1/2 cup butter, melted

Directions:
1. Fit the Breville Smart oven with the rack in position
2. In a mixing bowl, whisk eggs with milk, butter, crushed pineapple, and sugar.
3. Add bread cubes and stir well to coat.
4. Transfer mixture to the greased baking dish.
5. Set to bake at 350 F for 40 minutes. After 5 minutes place the baking dish in the preheated oven.
6. Serve and enjoy.
- **Nutrition Info:** Calories 510 Fat 17 g Carbohydrates 85 g Sugar 71 g Protein 3.4 g Cholesterol 123 mg

289. Cajun Sweet Potato Tots

Servings: 24
Cooking Time: 8 Minutes
Ingredients:
- 1/2 tsp Cajun seasoning
- 2 sweet potatoes, peeled
- Salt

Directions:
1. Fit the Breville Smart oven with the rack in position 2.
2. Add water in a large pot and bring to boil.
3. Add sweet potatoes to the pot and boil for 15 minutes. Drain well.
4. Grated boil sweet potatoes into a large bowl using a grated.
5. Add Cajun seasoning and salt in grated sweet potatoes and mix until well combined.
6. Make a small tot of sweet potato mixture and place in the air fryer basket then place an air fryer basket in the baking pan.
7. Place a baking pan on the oven rack. Set to air fry at 400 F for 8 minutes.
8. Serve and enjoy.

- **Nutrition Info:** Calories 10 Fat 0 g Carbohydrates 2.3 g Sugar 0 g Protein 0.1 g Cholesterol 0 mg

290. Cripsy Artichoke Bites

Servings: 4
Cooking Time: 8 Minutes
Ingredients:
- 14 whole artichoke hearts packed in water
- ½ cup all-purpose flour
- 1 egg
- $^1/_3$ cup panko bread crumbs
- 1 teaspoon Italian seasoning
- Cooking spray

Directions:
1. Drain the artichoke hearts and dry thoroughly with paper towels.
2. Place the flour on a plate. Beat the egg in a shallow bowl until frothy. Thoroughly combine the bread crumbs and Italian seasoning in a separate shallow bowl.
3. Dredge the artichoke hearts in the flour, then in the beaten egg, and finally roll in the bread crumb mixture until evenly coated.
4. Place the artichoke hearts in the air fryer basket and mist them with cooking spray.
5. Put the air fryer basket on the baking pan and slide into Rack Position 2, select Air Fry, set temperature to 375ºF (190ºC), and set time to 8 minutes.
6. Flip the artichoke hearts halfway through the cooking time.
7. When cooking is complete, the artichoke hearts should start to brown and the edges should be crispy. Remove from the oven and let the artichoke hearts sit for 5 minutes before serving.

291. French Apple Cake

Servings: 9
Cooking Time: 25 Minutes
Ingredients:
- 2 ¾ oz flour
- 5 tbsp sugar
- 1 ¼ oz butter
- 3 tbsp cinnamon
- 2 whole apple, sliced

Directions:

1. Preheat Breville Smart on Bake function to 360 F. In a bowl, mix 3 tbsp sugar, butter, and flour and form a pastry dough. Roll out the pastry on a floured surface and transfer it to the fryer's baking dish. Arrange the apple slices atop.
2. Cover the apples with sugar and cinnamon and cook for 20 minutes. Sprinkle with powdered sugar and mint and serve.

292.Crunchy Parmesan And Garlic Zucchini

Servings:x
Cooking Time:x
Ingredients:
- 1 cup panko crumbs, seasoned with salt, pepper and paprika
- 1 cup freshly grated parmesan
- 3 Tbsp olive oil
- 4-6 small green zucchini, sliced into spears by cutting into ½
- lengthwise and then into thirds
- Coarse salt and pepper, to taste
- 4 garlic cloves, sliced thin

Directions:
1. Preheat oven to 450°F.
2. Heat oil in a large Breville smart oven on medium-low heat.
3. Add zucchini and let brown on one side for 3 minutes and flip over pieces. Cook for another 3 minutes.
4. Sprinkle with salt and pepper.
5. Add sliced garlic and saute for 1 minute.
6. Sprinkle panko crumbs and grated cheese on top.
7. Transfer to oven until brown and bubbly, about 5-10 minutes.

293.Cappuccino Blondies

Servings: 16
Cooking Time: 30 Minutes
Ingredients:
- Nonstick cooking spray
- 1 cup butter, soft
- 2 cups brown sugar
- 2 eggs
- 2 tsp baking powder
- 1 tsp salt

- 4 tsp espresso powder
- 2 2/3 cups flour

Directions:
1. Place rack in position Lightly spray an 8x11-inch baking pan with cooking spray.
2. In a large bowl, beat together butter and sugar. Add eggs and beat until light and fluffy.
3. Add baking powder, salt, and espresso and mix well. Stir in flour until combined.
4. Set oven to bake on 350°F for 35 minutes.
5. Spread batter in prepared pan. Once oven has preheated, place brownies in oven and bake 25-30 minutes.
6. Remove from oven and let cool before cutting.
- **Nutrition Info:** Calories 296, Total Fat 12g, Saturated Fat 7g, Total Carbs 44g, Net Carbs 43g, Protein 3g, Sugar 28g, Fiber 1g, Sodium 254mg, Potassium 137mg, Phosphorus 82mg

294.Vanilla And Oats Pudding

Servings:x
Cooking Time:x
Ingredients:
- 2 tbsp. custard powder
- 3 tbsp. powdered sugar
- 3 tbsp. unsalted butter
- 2 cups vanilla powder
- 2 cups milk
- 1 cup oats

Directions:
1. Boil the milk and the sugar in a pan and add the custard powder followed by the vanilla powder followed by the oats and stir till you get a thick mixture.
2. Preheat the fryer to 300 Fahrenheit for five minutes. Place the dish in the basket and reduce the temperature to 250 Fahrenheit. Cook for ten minutes and set aside to cool.

295.Cheddar Dip

Servings: 6
Cooking Time: 15 Minutes
Ingredients:
- 8 oz. cheddar cheese; grated
- 12 oz. coconut cream

- 2 tsp. hot sauce

Directions:
1. In ramekin, mix the cream with hot sauce and cheese and whisk.
2. Put the ramekin in the fryer and cook at 390°F for 12 minutes. Whisk, divide into bowls and serve as a dip
- **Nutrition Info:** Calories: 170; Fat: 9g; Fiber: 2g; Carbs: 4g; Protein: 12g

296.Air Fryer Mixed Nuts

Servings: 2
Cooking Time: 4 Minutes
Ingredients:
- 2 cup mixed nuts
- 1 tbsp olive oil
- 1 tsp ground cumin
- 1 tsp pepper
- 1/4 tsp cayenne
- 1 tsp salt

Directions:
1. Fit the Breville Smart oven with the rack in position 2.
2. In a bowl, add all ingredients and toss well.
3. Add the nuts mixture to the air fryer basket then place an air fryer basket in the baking pan.
4. Place a baking pan on the oven rack. Set to air fry at 350 F for 4 minutes.
5. Serve and enjoy.
- **Nutrition Info:** Calories 953 Fat 88.2 g Carbohydrates 33.3 g Sugar 6.4 g Protein 22.7 g Cholesterol 0 mg

297.Vanilla Rum Cookies With Walnuts

Servings: 6
Cooking Time: 15 Minutes
Ingredients:
- 1/2 cup almond flour
- 1/2 cup coconut flour
- 1/2 teaspoon baking powder
- 1/4 teaspoon fine sea salt
- 1 stick butter, unsalted and softened
- 1/2 cup swerve
- 1 egg
- 1/2 teaspoon vanilla
- 1 teaspoon butter rum flavoring
- 3 ounces walnuts, finely chopped

Directions:
1. Begin by preheating the Air Fryer to 360 degrees F.
2. In a mixing dish, thoroughly combine the flour with baking powder and salt.
3. Beat the butter and swerve with a hand mixer until pale and fluffy; add the whisked egg, vanilla, and butter rum flavoring; mix again to combine well. Now, stir in the dry ingredients.
4. Fold in the chopped walnuts and mix to combine. Divide the mixture into small balls; flatten each ball with a fork and transfer them to a foil-lined baking pan.
5. Bake in the preheated Air Fryer for 14 minutes. Work in a few batches and transfer to wire racks to cool completely.
- **Nutrition Info:** 314 Calories; 32g Fat; 7g Carbs; 2g Protein; 2g Sugars; 5g Fiber

298.Choco Cookies

Servings: 8
Cooking Time: 8 Minutes
Ingredients:
- 3 egg whites
- 3/4 cup cocoa powder, unsweetened
- 1 3/4 cup confectioner sugar
- 1 1/2 tsp vanilla

Directions:
1. Fit the Breville Smart oven with the rack in position
2. In a mixing bowl, whip egg whites until fluffy soft peaks. Slowly add in cocoa, sugar, and vanilla.
3. Drop teaspoonful onto parchment-lined baking pan into 32 small cookies.
4. Set to bake at 350 F for 8 minutes. After 5 minutes place the baking pan in the preheated oven.
5. Serve and enjoy.
- **Nutrition Info:** Calories 132 Fat 1.1 g Carbohydrates 31 g Sugar 0.3 g Protein 2 g Cholesterol 0 mg

299.Keto Mixed Berry Crumble Pots

Servings: 6
Cooking Time: 15 Minutes
Ingredients:

- 2 ounces unsweetened mixed berries
- 1/2 cup granulated swerve
- 2 tablespoons golden flaxseed meal
- 1/4 teaspoon ground star anise
- 1/2 teaspoon ground cinnamon
- 1 teaspoon xanthan gum
- 2/3 cup almond flour
- 1 cup powdered swerve
- 1/2 teaspoon baking powder
- 1/3 cup unsweetened coconut, finely shredded
- 1/2 stick butter, cut into small pieces

Directions:
1. Toss the mixed berries with the granulated swerve, golden flaxseed meal, star anise, cinnamon, and xanthan gum. Divide between six custard cups coated with cooking spray.
2. In a mixing dish, thoroughly combine the remaining ingredients. Sprinkle over the berry mixture.
3. Bake in the preheated Air Fryer at 330 degrees F for 35 minutes. Work in batches if needed.

- **Nutrition Info:** 155 Calories; 13g Fat; 1g Carbs; 1g Protein; 8g Sugars; 6g Fiber

300.Orange Citrus Blend

Servings:x
Cooking Time:x
Ingredients:
- 3 tbsp. powdered sugar
- 3 tbsp. unsalted butter
- 2 oranges (sliced)
- 2 persimmons (sliced)
- 2 cups milk
- 2 cups almond flour
- 2 tbsp. custard powder

Directions:
1. Boil the milk and the sugar in a pan and add the custard powder followed by the almond flour and stir till you get a thick mixture. Add the sliced fruits to the mixture.
2. Preheat the fryer to 300 Fahrenheit for five minutes. Place the dish in the basket and reduce the temperature to 250 Fahrenheit. Cook for ten minutes and set aside to cool.

Printed in the USA
CPSIA information can be obtained
at www.ICGtesting.com
LVHW081815051224
798313LV00004B/582

* 9 7 8 1 8 0 1 2 4 5 4 6 3 *